Hospital Counselling and Rehabilitation Services

Hospital Counselling and Rehabilitation Services

C. Charles

ANMOL PUBLICATIONS PVT. LTD.
NEW DELHI - 110 002 (INDIA)

ANMOL PUBLICATIONS PVT. LTD.
H.O.: 4374/4B, Ansari Road, Daryaganj,
New Delhi-110 002 (India)
Ph.: 23278000, 23261597
B.O.: No. 1015, Ist Main Road, BSK IIIrd Stage
IIIrd Phase, IIIrd Block,
Bangalore - 560 085 (India)
Visit us at: www.anmolpublications.com

Hospital Counselling and Rehabilitation Services

First Published, 2008

ISBN 978-81-261-3290-4

PRINTED IN INDIA

Printed at Mehra Offset Press, Delhi.

Contents

Preface

This publication entitled "Hospital Counseling and Rehabilitation Services" is published specifically to clarify the business, medical and operational aspects of hospital counseling and rehabilitation services in the modern age. The focus lies on key issues, including convincing about innovative medical technologies, patient care and medical treatments. Medical counseling on the computer communication network is being used increasingly with wide-ranging concern of people about health and strengthening the role of medical care as social service. This book explores main problems/issues of network counseling and to suggest future prosperity of medical counseling. Inquiry about symptoms is the most common reason for encounter, followed by treatment and prevention strategies, detailed information about diseases, and inquiry about laboratory tests. Systematic classification showed common problems of skin, digestive, musculo-skeletal and general & unspecified, which was a different look compared with common problems in primary care. The answer content presents a different look among various groups. Common answers are mainly to offer medical information, to recommend visiting a doctor, and to provide self-care remedies. Network counseling supplements the incompleteness of medical interview with doctors, and make it easy to communicate various pieces of information between patients and doctors. Counseling psychology is the branch of psychology that focuses on personal problems not classified as serious mental disorders, such as academic, social, or vocational difficulties of students. This is similar to clinical psychology, except that most of the issues addressed by counseling psychologists are less serious. For example, a clinical psychologist would be more likely to deal with schizophrenia and other serious psychological disorders than a counseling psychologist. Bereavement counseling is assistance and support to people with emotional and psychological stress after the death of a loved one. Bereavement counseling includes a broad range of transition services, including outreach, counseling, and referral services to family members.

A licensed clinical professional counselor is a mental health professional trained in the application of psychotherapy techniques. The main focus of their work is to improvement the quality of life and life choices a person makes. A major goal is broadening possible decisions and helping to determine new alternatives for old behaviors and feelings which may have caused emotional discomfort. Counselors can work with friends, family, and the person who's going through it. Coping and healing involves refocusing their lives, understanding abilities and limitations, moving through stages of loss, and coming out the other side finding new ways to feel good about themselves and their life. There are many strategies counselors use to help people heal and move forward. There are two levels of counselors. The first level requires supervision from another licensed professional, while the second level can practice independently and diagnosis and treat mental and emotional disorders.

Rehabilitation implies a comprehensive program for patients to follow to reduce or overcome deficits following injury or illness. They assist the individual to gain the optimal mental and physical ability. Rehabilitation Psychology is the helping profession dedicated to assisting people—individuals, family members, and caregivers—who are struggling with the effects of a disability and are seeking to restore hope and meaning to their lives. Nearly one in five Americans has a disability. Every age, cultural and gender group is affected. Disability refers to a limitation in physical, sensory, cognitive (thinking), or emotional functioning. A disability can affect a person's capacity to work, to learn, to manage personal or family responsibilities, to maintain relationships, or to participate in recreational activities. Examples of some of the most common conditions resulting in disability are: spinal cord injury, stroke, brain injury, multiple sclerosis, cerebral palsy, Parkinson's Disease, cancer, diabetes, amputation, Alzheimer's Disease, orthopedic injury, learning disability, pervasive developmental disorders, vision and hearing impairment, arthritis, and pain syndromes. To become specialists in the care of people affected by disabilities, Rehabilitation Psychologists must complete a doctoral degree in psychology and an internship or other, focused, intensive training program in which they acquire experience serving people with a wide range of disabilities. The services provided by Rehabilitation Psychologists include: assessment; counseling; compensatory strategies; wellness promotion; stress management for caregivers; education and consultation to involved community members, such as employers or teachers; and referrals to other specialists when needed. Rehabilitation Psychologists are the specialists trained and dedicated to helping people affected by a disability succeed in reclaiming their sense of belonging, of contribution, of value, and of meaningful participation in the world. Drug rehabilitation (often shortened to drug rehab or just rehab) is an umbrella term for the processes of medical and/or psychotherapeutic treatment, for dependency on psychoactive substances such as alcohol, prescription drugs , and so-called street drugs such as cocaine, heroin or amphetamines. The obvious intent is to enable the patient to cease their previous level of abuse, for the sake of avoiding its psychological, legal, social, and physical consequences, especially in extreme abuse. Drug rehabilitation tends to address the two fold nature of drug dependency; physical and psychological dependency. Physical dependency involves a detoxification process to cope with withdrawal symptoms from regular use of a drug. With regular use of many drugs, legal or otherwise, the brain gradually adapts to the presence of the drug so that normal functioning can occur. This is how physical tolerance develops to drugs such as heroin, amphetamines, cocaine, nicotine or alcohol. It is also why more of the drug is needed to get the same effect with regular use. The abrupt cessation of taking a drug can lead to withdrawal symptoms where the body may take weeks, to possibly months (depending on the drug involved) before things get back to normal. Psychological dependency is addressed in many drug rehabilitation programs by attempting to teach the patient new methods of interacting in a drug free method. In particular, patients are generally encouraged or required not to associate with friends who still use the addictive substance. Twelve-step programs encourage addicts not only to stop using alcohol or other drugs, but to examine and change habits related to their addictions. Many programs emphasize that recovery is a permanent process without a culmination. For legal drugs such as alcohol complete abstention rather than attempts at moderation, which may lead to relapse are also emphasized ("One drink is too many; one hundred drinks is not enough.") Whether moderation is achievable by persons with a history of abuse remains a controversial point but is generally considered unsustainable. There are various types of programs that offer help in drug rehabilitation, including: residential treatment (in-patient), out-patient, local support groups, extended care centers, and sober houses.

Pharmacotherapies to a greater or lesser extent have come to play a part in drug rehabilitation. Medications such as methadone and more recently buprenorphine are widely used and show significant efficacy in the treatment of opioid dependence, that is to drugs such as heroin, morphine or oxycontin. Methadone and buprenorphine are maintenance therapies used with an intent of stabilizing an abnormal opioid system and used for long durations of time though both may be used to withdraw patients from narcotics over short term periods as well. Ibogaine, an experimental medication is proposed to interrupt both physical dependence and psychological craving to a broad range or drugs including narcotics, stimulants, alcohol and nicotine. Some antidepressants also show use in moderating drug use particularly to nicotine and it has become common for researchers to reexamine already approved drugs for new uses in drug rehabilitation. Drug rehabilitation is sometimes part of the criminal justice system. People convicted of minor drug offenses may be sentenced to rehabilitation instead of prison, and those convicted of driving while intoxicated are sometimes required to attend Alcoholics Anonymous meetings. Rehabilitation of sensory and cognitive function typically involves methods for retraining neural pathways or training new neural pathways to regain or improve neurocognitive functioning that has been diminished by disease or traumatic injury.

This publication entitled "Hospital Counseling and Rehabilitation Services" covers most of the issues related to contemporary global and national developments in the said field.

—Editor

1

Hospital Counselling and Rehabilitation Services: An Introduction

SUPERVISION OF GROUP COUNSELLORS

Quality supervision is important because it provides support to the group drug counsellor, helps him or her develop skills, and ensures that counsellors adhere to the treatment protocol. Not all counsellors will require the same amount of supervision, with more experienced counsellors likely to require less intensive supervision. However, accountability is important, no matter how experienced the counsellor is. The programme of supervision described in this study was used with therapists in the NIDA-supported multisite treatment project from which the efficacy data came (e.g., Crits-Christoph et al. 1999). It is strongly recommended that counsellors participate in a regular programme of supervision that assesses how well they adhere to this treatment model. Supervision as part of the research protocol involved videotaping each GDC session, having supervisors rate selected sessions on adherence to the therapeutic model, and discussing clinical issues and adherence with counsellors. Supervision sessions took place weekly until counsellors demonstrated consistently that they could adhere to the model, and then these sessions occurred every other week.

Supervisors used an adherence scale to rate counsellors' adherence to the therapeutic model, both for videotaped sessions viewed regularly and for an overall yearly review. The adherence scale contains three general categories of therapist strategies—Supporting Recovery, Encouraging 12-Step Participation, and Facilitating Group Participation—and a fourth category specific to either a Phase I or Phase II group session. Supporting Recovery strategies include encouraging clients to abstain from substance use and to discuss episodes of use or cravings, and giving clients feedback about their progress in recovery. Encouraging 12-Step Participation involves expressing positive opinions about the 12-Step approach, encouraging attendance at meetings, and reciting the Serenity Prayer aloud with group members. Facilitating Group Participation includes encouraging group members to give each other constructive feedback and positive reinforcement, and creating an atmosphere of trust and confidentiality. For Phase I and II group sessions, counsellor adherence is rated based on the degree to which counsellors facilitated group progress, with Phase I group sessions requiring more structure than Phase II group sessions.

COUNSELLING

Health and Social Services offer a free, private and confidential counselling service.

When?

Sometimes we may experience feelings which cause distress or which we are unable to control, like loss or anger. Some people find that they are unable to cope with these emotions and cannot move on. Counselling is there to enable you to make progress. When a sudden crisis is experienced, don't bottle up your feelings. Counselling can help you strengthen your coping skills.

Why?

There are those times when the assistance of a qualified counsellor/therapist can be very supportive in listening to your problems/concerns. Counselling can help you make some sense of what is happening to you, and to give you support at these difficult periods in your life.

If you have any of the signs below then consider contacting Anne:

— Loneliness
— Depression and sadness
— Feelings of failure, stress, anxiety
— Problems with anger, being out of control
— Panic or anxiety
— Problems with alcohol or drugs
— Feelings of loss or grief
— Problems following an accident
— Problems relating to work
— Issues following bereavement

How can I see Anne Lane?

The Hospital Counsellor - Anne Lane has been in post for several years. She is a member of the UK Register of Counsellors, and abides by the British Association of Counselling Code of ethics and confidentiality. She is Counsellor for staff, patients and relatives.

If you would like to talk to Anne please ask the nurse caring for you to contact her to make an appointment. You will be able to talk privately. Anne is also available for relatives if they have any anxieties they wish to share, again in privacy and in confidence.

Anne sees patients in the wards, and also in her rooms when people are discharged if this is required by the patient.

What Anne Cannot do for You

Anne is not a social worker, and cannot, for example advise on housing benefits.

Anne is not a Psychiatrist.

Anne will not tell you what to do.

What Anne can do for you

She is here to listen to your concerns and to help you understand your feelings. Counselling can give back to people a feeling of being able to make their own choices in the future. In a situation which cannot be changed then the change exits in adjusting to new circumstances.

Sharing experiences with a Counsellor can be a tremendous relief. Counselling can help you to make sense of what is happening in your life.

PSYCHOEDUCATIONAL GROUP SESSIONS

Phase I is a structured, psychoeducational group that is offered for 90 minutes per session for the first 12 weeks of treatment. The psycho-educational group is designed to enhance knowledge regarding addiction and recovery. During this early period in recovery, many cocaine-dependent clients experience postacute withdrawal symptoms, struggle with their motivation to change, and are only beginning to abstain from cocaine and other substances. Therefore, they need support and encouragement in addition to information about addiction and recovery.

Purpose

Phase I group sessions are designed to provide clients with relatively frequent, supportive contact with the counsellor and other men and women in recovery; introduce clients to key concepts about addiction and the recovery process; help clients understand how they may set themselves up to relapse; and help clients develop strategies to reduce their relapse risk. The group programme helps empower members to establish and maintain abstinence, develop a sense of personal responsibility for their recovery, develop supportive interpersonal relationships, and continue participating in a self-help programme such as AA, NA, CA, or other support groups.

Weekly Group Topics

Each weekly Phase I group session focuses on one of the following recovery topics:

— Session #1: Symptoms of Cocaine Addiction

— Session #2: The Process of Recovery: Part I

— Session #3: The Process of Recovery: Part II

— Session #4: Managing Cravings: People, Places, and Things

— Session #5: Relationships in Recovery

— Session #6: Self-Help Groups

— Session #7: Establishing a Support System

— Session #8: Managing Feelings in Recovery

— Session #9: Coping With Guilt and Shame

— Session #10 Warning Signs of Relapse

— Session #11: Coping With High-Risk Situations

— Session #12: Maintaining Recovery

Format of Phase I Psychoeducational Group Sessions

1. Check-in period: At the beginning of each group session, clients introduce themselves by stating their names, admitting that they are addicted to cocaine (and other substances, if relevant), indicating the last day they used addictive substances, and briefly discussing strong cravings, close calls, or actual episodes of drug use. This usually lasts 10 to 20 minutes.

2. *Review of session topic and objectives:* The group counsellor briefly introduces the topic and the objectives of the group session so that members have an idea of the specific issues that will be covered. The group counsellor passes out handouts to group members and asks them to complete the checklists or answer the questions on these handouts. This usually takes about 10 minutes.

3. *Review of curriculum and members' responses to questions on handouts:* The group counsellor introduces the topic and objectives for the session and leads the group in a discussion of the topic. Group members are encouraged to share their experiences, and the group counsellor attempts to highlight the connection between group members' input and the identified topic.

4. *Review of the plan for the upcoming week:* The group counsellor asks each member to briefly state what actions he or she plans to take in the upcoming week in his or her recovery from cocaine addiction. Group members can mention self-help meetings they plan to attend and other steps they will take in their recovery. This usually takes 5 to 15 minutes.

5. *Reciting the Serenity Prayer:* The group ends after members join hands and say the Serenity Prayer out loud. The Serenity Prayer states: "God, grant me the serenity to accept the things I cannot change, the courage to change the things I can, and the wisdom to know the difference." After the prayer, the leader encourages all members to return for the group session next week.

Strategies for Covering Group Curriculum

Since the therapy groups are small, consisting of fewer than 10 clients, it is preferable to cover the educational curriculum interactively by involving the group members. However, the leader can give "mini-lectures" by presenting particular issues or points in an educational way during the course of the GDC session. The group counsellor should refrain, however, from spending too much time lecturing. While information on addiction and recovery is important, mutual support, sharing one's own experiences, and discussing clients' reactions to the material are also important in GDC sessions. Often the most effective teaching is done in an interactive format because clients learn most from what they think about and contribute in the group.

COUNSELLING AND DISCHARGE FROM HOSPITAL

The discharge process for all children should include:

- correct timing of discharge from hospital
- counselling the mother on treatment and feeding of the child at home
- ensuring that the child's immunisation status and record card are up-to-date
- communicating with the health worker who referred the child or who will beresponsible for follow-up care
- instructions on when to return to the hospital for follow-up and on symptomsand signs indicating the need to return urgently
- assisting the family with special support (e.g. providing equipment for achild with a disability, or linking with community support organisations forchildren with HIV/AIDS).

Timing of Discharge from Hospital

In general, in the management of acute infections, the child can be consideredready for discharge after the clinical condition has improved markedly (afebrile,alert, eating and sleeping normally) and oral treatment has been started.Decisions on when to discharge should be made on an individual basis, takinginto consideration a number of factors, such as:

— the family's home circumstances and how much support is available to carefor the child
— the staff's judgement of the likelihood that the family will return immediatelyto the hospital if the child's condition should worsen.

Timing of discharge of the child with severe malnutrition is particularlyimportant and is discussed separately discussed in this study. In every case,the family should be given as much warning as possible of the discharge dateso that appropriate arrangements can be made to support the child at home.If the family removes the child prematurely against the advice of the hospitalstaff, counsel the mother on how to continue treatment at home and encourageher to bring the child for follow-up after 1–2 days, and to make contact withthe local health worker for help in the follow-up care of the child.

Nutrition Counselling

Identifying feeding problems

First, identify any feeding problems which have not been fully resolved.

Ask the following questions:

— Do you breastfeed your child?
— How many times during the day?

— Do you also breastfeed during the night?
— Does the child take any other food or fluids?
— What food or fluids?
— How many times a day?
— What do you use to feed the child?
— How large are the servings?
— Does the child receive his/her own serving?
— Who feeds the child and how?

Compare the child's actual feeding with the recommended guidelines for feedinga child of that age. Identify any differences andlist these as feeding problems.

In addition to the issues addressed above, consider:

— Difficulty in breastfeeding
— Use of a feeding bottle
— Lack of active feeding
— Not feeding well during the illness

Advise the mother how to overcome problems and how to feed the child.

Refer to local feeding recommendations for children of different ages. Theserecommendations should include details of locally appropriate energy-rich andnutrient-rich complementary foods.

Even when specific feeding problems are not found, praise the mother forwhat she does well. Give her advice that promotes:

— breastfeeding
— improved complementary feeding practices using locally availableenergy- and nutrient-rich foods

— the giving of nutritious snacks to children aged =2 years.

Counselling

Mother's Card

A simple, pictorial card reminding the mother of home care instructions, whento return for follow-up care, and the signs indicating the need to returnimmediately to the hospital can be given to each mother. This Mother's Cardwill help her to remember the appropriate foods and fluids, and when to returnto the health worker.Appropriate Mother's Cards are being developed as part of local training forIntegrated Management of Childhood Illness (IMCI). Check first whether onehas been produced in your area and use that. For details of where to find an example.When reviewing the Mother's Card with the mother:

— Hold the card so that she can easily see the pictures, or allow her to hold itherself

— Point to the pictures as you talk, and explain each one; this will help her toremember what the pictures represent.

— Mark the information that is relevant to the mother. For example, put a circleround the feeding advice for the child's age, and round the signs to returnimmediately. If the child has diarrhoea, tick the appropriate fluid(s) to begiven. Record the date for the next immunisation.

— Watch to see if the mother looks worried or puzzled. If so, encouragequestions.

— Ask the mother to tell you in her own words what she should do at home.Encourage her to use the card to help her remember.

— Give her the card to take home. Suggest she show it

to other family members.(If you do not have a large enough supply of cards to give to every mother,keep several in the clinic to show to mothers.)

Home Treatment

— Use words the mother understands.

— Use teaching aids that are familiar (e.g. common containers for mixing ORS).

— Allow the mother to practise what she must do, e.g. preparing ORS solutionor giving an oral medication, and encourage her to ask questions.

— Give advice in a helpful and constructive manner, praising the mother forcorrect answers or good practice.

Teaching mothers is not just about giving instructions. It should include thefollowing steps:

— Give information. Explain to the mother how to give the treatment, e.g.preparing ORS, giving an oral antibiotic, or applying eye ointment.

— Show an example. Show the mother how to give the treatment by demon-strating what to do.

— Let her practise. Ask the mother to prepare the medicine or give thetreatment while you watch her. Help her as needed, so that she does itcorrectly.

— Check her understanding.

Ask the mother to repeat the instructions in herown words, or ask her questions to see that she has understood correctly.

Checking Immunisation Status

Ask to see the child's immunisation card, and determine whether all the immunisations recommended for the child's age have been given. Note anyimmunisations the child still needs and explain this to the mother; then carrythem out before the child leaves hospital and record them on the card.

Checking the Mother's Own Health

If the mother is sick, provide treatment for her and help to arrange follow-upat a first-level clinic close to her home. Check the mother's nutritional statusand give any appropriate counselling. Check the mother's immunisation statusand, if needed, give her tetanus toxoid. Make sure the mother has access tofamily planning and counselling about preventing sexually-transmitted diseasesand HIV. If the child has tuberculosis, the mother should have a chest X-ray and Mantoux test. Make sure the mother knows where to have them and explainwhy they are needed.

Contraindications

It is important to immunize all children, including those who are sick and mal-nourished, unless there are contraindications. There are only 3 contra-indications to immunisation:

- Do not give BCG or yellow fever vaccines to a child with symptomatic HIVinfection/AIDS, but do give the other vaccines.
- Give all immunisations, including BCG and yellow fever vaccines, to a childwith asymptomatic HIV infection.
- Do not give DPT-2 or -3 to a child who has had convulsions or shock within 3 days of the most recent dose.
- Do not give DPT to a child with recurrent convulsions or an activeneurological disease of the central nervous system.

A child with diarrhoea who is due to receive OPV should be given a dose of OPV. However, this dose should not be counted in the schedule. Make a noteon the child's immunisation record that it coincided with diarrhoea, so that thehealth worker will know this and give the child an extra dose.

Communicating with the First-level Health Worker

Information Needed

The first-level health worker who referred the child to hospital should receiveinformation about the child's care in hospital, which should include:

- — diagnosis/diagnoses
- — treatment(s) given (and duration of stay in hospital)
- — response of the child to this treatment
- — instructions given to the mother for follow-up treatment or other care athome
- — other matters for follow-up (e.g. immunisations).

If the child has a health card, the above information can be recorded on it andthe mother should be requested to show this to the health worker. Where thereis no health card, these details should be recorded in a short note for themother and health worker.

Follow-up for feeding and nutritional problems

- — If a child has a feeding problem and you have recommended changes infeeding, follow up in 5 days to see if the mother has made the changes, andgive further counselling if needed.
- — If a child has anaemia, follow up in 14 days to give more oral iron.
- — If the child has a very low weight, additional follow-

up is needed in 30 days.This follow-up would involve weighing the child, reassessing feedingpractices, and giving further nutritional counselling.

When to return immediately

Advise the mother to return immediately if the child develops any of the follow-ing signs:

— not able to drink or breastfeed

— becomes sicker

— develops a fever

— signs of illness return again after successful treatment in hospital

— in a child with a cough or cold: fast or difficult breathing

— in a child with diarrhoea: blood in stool or drinking poorly.

Next well-child Visit

Remind the mother about the child's next visit for immunisation and recordthe date on the Mother's Card or the child's immunisation record.

Providing Follow-up Care

Children who do not require hospital admission but can be treated at homeAdvise all mothers who are taking their children home, after assessment in thehospital, when to go to a health worker for follow-up care. Mothers may needto return to hospital:

— for a follow-up visit in a specific number of days (e.g. when it is necessaryto check progress or the response to an antibiotic)

— if signs appear that suggest the illness is worsening

— for the child's next immunisation.

It is especially important to teach the mother the signs indicating the need toreturn to hospital immediately. Guidance on the follow-up of specific clinicalconditions is given in appropriate sections of this pocket book.

2

Role of Adviser and Informed Consent

EDUCATIONAL TECHNIQUES USED IN CHANGING PROVIDER BEHAVIOUR

A number of techniques have been used to modify the behaviour of practicing physicians. Continuing medical education, practice guidelines and critical pathways represent a major thrust of these efforts. The relative effectiveness of each is largely dependent on the particular strategy employed in their implementation. Traditionally these strategies have focused on lectures and printed materials but other techniques have also been utilized, including audit and feedback, academic detailing, local opinion leaders and reminder systems. In addition, some have championed the use of sentinel event reporting and root cause analysis in graduate medical education programmes. Only recently have these various techniques been critically evaluated for their effectiveness at changing physician behaviour.

Prevalence and Severity of Target Safety Problem/ Opportunities for Impact

It is well established that physicians are unable to keep abreast of the staggering volume of published medical literature. This is reflected by the many studies that demonstrate the glacial pace at which many beneficial advances are incorporated into medical practice. Practice guidelines, clinical decision support systems and programmes for physician education are potential solutions to this problem, but their effectiveness is greatly dependent on the methods used in their implementation. Despite the presence of comprehensive guidelines on the treatment of reactive airways disease, for example, a substantial percentage of asthmatic patients do not receive appropriate care. Physician education techniques that reliably impact practice patterns may yield substantial improvements in patient care and safety.

Practice Description

The passive dissemination of information through the use of lectures, conferences, mailings and printed materials remains the primary method to alter physician behaviour. This primacy has not been substantially challenged in practice, although more interactive techniques have increasingly been utilized. *Academic detailing*, for example, involves the process of having invested and well-informed agents for change interacting with individual physicians to promote certain tenets of practice.

Alternatively, *audit and feedback* entails the review and return to the clinician of their own process of care and patient outcomes (often compared with local or national benchmarks or evidence-based standards) in the hopes it will result in more appropriate medical care. *Reminder systems*, which may be computerized and embedded in the electronic medical record, prompt physicians to provide certain healthcare measures. They differ from *clinical decision support systems* in that they may not provide information tailored to the specific patient. Finally, *opinion leaders*, usually respected local physicians, may improve healthcare by championing "best practices" on a regional basis.

Study Outcomes

Few of the studies report outcomes specific to the field of patient safety. The vast majority are concerned with process of care rather than the outcomes of care. Although clinical outcomes are reported in at least one of the studies evaluated in each of the systematic reviews (with one exception), the majority relate outcomes pertaining to physician performance. Some of the more commonly described variables include the rates of appropriate provision of preventive care measures and of adherence to appropriate treatment or diagnostic protocols.

Study Designs

The Cochrane Group completed a series of systematic reviews of physician education based on the Research and Development Base in Continuing Medical Education, a central database compiled from an extensive search of electronic databases and bibliographies and supplemented by contact with experts in the field. Although the initial review was completed in 1997, reviews are regularly updated as more pertinent data are published. One such study evaluated the role of audit and feedback and found 37 randomized controlled studies comparing this technique to non-interventional control groups.

An ancillary study by the Cochrane Group compared audit and feedback with other educational strategies and located 12 randomized controlled studies for analysis. A second study of the effectiveness of audit and feedback was completed by a separate group that searched MEDLINE and selected bibliographies for trials investigating the strategy's utility in improving immunization rates. Fifteen studies were identified for inclusion, 5 of which were randomized controlled studies with 6 interrupted time series evaluations and 4 before-after trials. A third meta-analysis of peer-comparison feedback systems used an extensive electronic database and bibliography search to locate 12 randomized controlled studies.

The Cochrane Group also investigated the utility of academic detailing and found 18 randomized controlled studies. A similar evaluation of local opinion leaders yielded 8 randomized controlled trials. A separate Cochrane review was completed on the utility of printed educational materials using the Cochrane Effective Practice and Organisation of Care Group database. The search of this database, which was compiled in the same manner as the Research and Development Base in Continuing Medical Education, found 10 randomized controlled trials and one interrupted time series study fulfilling criteria for analysis.

Evidence for Effectiveness of Practice

Much of the evidence for the effectiveness of educational and implementation techniques is of fair quality and the results are generally consistent across the various systematic reviews. However, methodologic concerns prevented the completion of quantitative data synthesis in the majority of the reviews. The initial comprehensive review found overall beneficial effect for 62% of interventions. In investigations of effect on patient outcomes, 48% had favourable results. Academic detailing and the use of local opinion leaders were the most effective techniques evaluated. Physician reminder systems were also effective, as 22 of the 26 evaluated studies revealed some benefit. The technique of audit and feedback was of marginal effectiveness and conferences and printed materials were found to be relatively ineffective. Of note, multifaceted interventions with at least 3 components were associated with a 71% success rate. The second comprehensive review of 102 randomized controlled studies supported these conclusions. Yet it emphasized that the degree of effect with even the most consistently effective techniques was moderate at best, and that the process of care rather than the outcome of care was the most readily influenced variable.

The Cochrane reviews reported similar results. Audit and feedback was found to be effective in 62% of the studies in which it was compared with non-interventional controls, but the effect was typically small. The results were not substantially different when audit and feedback was augmented by conferences or educational materials or was part of a multifaceted intervention. In the review of comparative trials, however, this technique was found to be inferior to reminder systems in 2 of the 3 trials where a direct comparison was made. The second review of audit and feedback, which focused on improving immunization rates, found beneficial results in 4 of 5 randomized controlled trials evaluated. Statistically significant changes were present in at least 2 of these evaluations. However, the marginal effect was small and likely was overwhelmed by the relatively high cost of the intervention. Finally the meta-analysis of the 12 randomized controlled trials investigating peer-comparison feedback systems did establish a modest benefit for the use of audit and feedback ($p<0.05$), but the magnitude of benefit was again noted to be small. The Cochrane review of academic detailing was somewhat more optimistic. All of the evaluated studies showed some degree of a beneficial effect on physician performance although only one of these studies reported patient outcomes. Most combined detailing with other techniques and there was insufficient evidence to make direct comparisons between detailing and the other techniques.

The use of local opinion leaders was also found to be effective by the Cochrane group, although to a much less convincing degree than academic detailing. Two of 7 trials showed a statistically significant beneficial effect with a trend toward effectiveness in all 7 studies. One of 3 trials investigating patient outcomes demonstrated a significant benefit.

Finally, the Cochrane review of the use of printed educational materials supported the findings of the previous overviews. None of the 9 studies showed a statistically significant effect when compared with controls and only one of 6 trials that included printed materials in a multifaceted approach demonstrated benefit. Of note, all of the evaluated trials were plagued by methodologic shortcomings.

Potential for Harm

These educational techniques are unlikely to cause significant patient harm.

Comment

From studies of randomized controlled trials, it appears that academic detailing and local opinion leaders are frequently associated with at least some benefit. Reminder systems are also effective in specific situations and the utility of audit and feedback has been established, although unimpressively. Traditional programmes of conferences, lectures and printed materials are ineffective at inducing changes in physician behaviour. None of the current techniques, however, have demonstrated a consistent ability to induce substantial and durable changes in physician behaviour. The relative cost-effectiveness of the various techniques is uncertain; it remains unclear if the added cost of the more effective strategies (i.e., academic detailing and local opinion leaders) is justified given their relatively small marginal increase in effectiveness. Finally there are few data regarding the specific utility of these techniques in increasing patient safety and/or the prevention of medical errors. However, techniques effective in other areas of medicine are likely to be equally effective in inducing practices changes to improve patient safety.

Costs and Implementation

Although the cost-effectiveness of the various educational techniques has not been explicitly studied, it is clear that several may require substantial outlay in terms of financial resources and personnel. It also appears that the forms of education that are most effective, including academic detailing and local opinion leaders, are also the most expensive to design and support. Programmes of printed materials and lectures, although dramatically less effective, are substantially less expensive to implement. It is unclear whether the integration of Internet technology and computer-based education initiatives will result in substantial changes in efficacy or cost. Finally, the relative cost-effectiveness of the various techniques remains unclear.

MEDICAL ADVICE

AHA Legal Position

American Heart Association staff do *not* give personal medical advice or answer personal medical questions. Qualified staff in the Office of Science Operations at our National Center can answer scientific questions. National Center, affiliate and division staff are allowed to offer the association's official policy or statement about a given medical issue. The association cannot make referrals to physicians, cardiac surgeons, nurses, physicians assistants, nutritionists, physical therapists or occupational therapists. We can't maintain current information on whether such persons meet professional criteria across the wide variety of medical disciplines and geographic regions. Nor can we know enough about an individual's medical history, healthcare needs, financial or insurance situation to make proper referrals.

You can get such information from your local medical association or society.

Our association does not provide recommendations to individuals seeking healthcare sites, health maintenance organisations, hospitals, clinics or cardiac rehabilitation centers. We can't maintain current information on whether such places around the country meet accepted medical standards. Nor can we know enough about an individual's personal medical history, healthcare needs, financial or insurance situation to make proper referrals. You can get such information from your local health department or medical association or society. We also do not provide testimony or legal opinions to litigants in medical malpractice cases.

BEREAVEMENT ADVISER

In the late 1980s and early 1990s cardiac social workers provided a 24-hour on call service in the Alder Hey Cardiac Department and would sit with bereaved parents and talk to them. Clinicians would often take their lead from the cardiac social workers in terms of when the parents were able to cope with being given the necessary information following their child's death. The system worked very well and in the mid-1990s the cardiac social workers were replaced by cardiac liaison nurses. The service now is equally as good as the system it replaced. There is always a cardiac liaison nurse available for consultation at Alder Hey. There is also a community-based cardiac liaison nurse supported by the British Heart Foundation who is available to speak to parents at any time. In evidence the parents identified the need for this type of service. It should not be restricted to the cardiac department, but should be generally available. In his Interim Guidance on Post Mortem Examination issued on 1 March 2000 the Chief Medical Officer indicated that all NHS Hospital Trusts should designate a named individual in a Trust who will be available to provide support and information to families of the deceased where post mortem examination may be required, whether this is requested by a hospital doctor or the Coroner. This person should be trained in the management of bereavement. We feel that a bereavement adviser would be the person to discharge this role. Parents must be involved in decision-making as well as in requesting and accepting support. The aim is to assist them in the difficult period following death. Their individual feelings and needs must be identified and respected. Their paramount need is for accurate, consistent, co-ordinated information.

Choices available to parents should be fully explained, with all the necessary information provided. They must be given time together and time with their child. Time must also be available to make practical arrangements. They must be treated with respect and dignity at all times. The bereavement adviser should not be judgmental in dealing with parents. Parents must be supplied with clear, factual, unbiased information. Confusion must be avoided. Parents may need help with thinking what they want to ask and even asking their clinician questions. No subject should be avoided and they must be treated with honesty even if the truth is painful. Their confidentiality must be respected at all times. The bereavement adviser should try and ensure that parents are dealt with on equal terms by the clinician and other professionals and time must be made available to meet the parents' needs.

It should be understood that grief can be expressed differently in different cultures. The nature of grief is personal and private. In a hospital, which often appears impersonal and public, there should be a private place where the bereavement adviser and parents can meet and have time together or alone. Parents must have time, space and support to relive, think and talk about what has happened to them.

The training of a bereavement adviser should include the appropriate use of language, the need to provide individual attention and to anticipate the requirements of bereaved relatives. They must have a full understanding of post mortem procedures and the issue of consent. This will include identifying and distinguishing between a Coroner‘s and hospital post mortem examinations. They should be able to obtain information from clinicians and pathologists about the identification of organs to be retained and whether or not they will be retained beyond the funeral. Training must include why certain organs have to be “fixed‘ before examination and the length of time necessary to “fix‘ and examine a particular organ. The bereavement adviser must be able to advise on all aspects of the funeral including return of organs to the body following post mortem examination, or identification of organs, tissue, blocks, slides, X-rays and photographs retained beyond the funeral. An awareness of all funeral procedures, religious requirements and the purpose of memorial services is necessary.

There will be a psychological component in bereavement advisers‘ training, relating to sensitive and respectful communication as well as gentle treatment of stressful topics such as consent to post mortem procedure. They will require liaison skills in order to discuss matters with clinicians, Coroners and other professionals. The bereavement adviser should try to involve the pathologist more openly with clinicians and parents. The pathologist will be of particular assistance with regard to explaining why organs are retained and what purposes, including therapeutic, medical education and research, are served by retention of organs or tissue.

Parents should be given every opportunity to express their wishes about the eventual disposal of organs. A bereavement adviser can facilitate this. Parents' wishes must be respected. The need for respect cannot be overstated.

Every hospital should have a bereavement adviser. A dedicated office should be provided and include a private sitting area for parents or surviving relatives.

Recommendations

We have considered the evidence and recommend that the functions of a bereavement adviser include:

— Explaining the circumstances of death, identifying when, where and who was present.

— Arranging and attending a meeting for relatives with anyone who was present at the death if requested.

— Encouraging a meeting between relatives and the treating clinician to explain the clinical circumstances of death and if requested arranging and attending the meeting.

— Ensuring that relatives have a full explanation of the reasons for post mortem examination including therapeutic, medical education and research.

— Explaining the need for consent to carry out a hospital post mortem examination (HPM) and the retention of organs.

— Explaining that consent is necessary for the retention of organs following a Coroner's post mortem examination (CPM) and that the consent must be obtained before the CPM is undertaken.

— Ensuring relatives have sufficient time, privacy and support to reflect upon the request for consent to an HPM or the retention of organs following a CPM or an HPM.

— Ascertaining whether the clinician will attend post mortem examination.

— Facilitating meetings between parents, clinician and pathologist as appropriate.

— Noting discussions between relatives, clinicians and pathologists and providing a copy to each party involved.

— Developing and using information packs for relatives on all aspects of death in hospital.

— Assisting relatives in the following practical matters:

- collecting the deceased's personal belongings and arranging return to relatives; œ ensuring provision of certificate of death and the formal notice;
- explaining the procedure to register the death;
- providing support in attending the registry office if requested;
- arranging contact with funeral director;
- arranging contact with hospital chaplain and/or local priest as required;
- contacting the Coroner's office as appropriate;
- offering to attend if contact with police necessary;
- ensuring that the General Practitioner is informed;
- ensuring that schools are informed as appropriate (including the schools of siblings);
- assisting the relatives in informing other persons, including other relatives, friends and employers, of the death and its consequences;

  - assisting the relatives in dealing with the Benefits Agency, insurance company, housing matters;
  - assisting the relatives to place announcements in newspapers if wished.

- Discussing counselling or long-term support needs with relatives, including the needs of wider family members and making contact with appropriate counselling/support agencies if requested.
- Ensuring that relatives are aware of the full range of counselling/support resources available including those external to the hospital and bringing these matters to the attention of the relatives.
- Accessing translation/interpreting services including services for people with hearing or visual impairment and providing appropriate written/taped information.
- Assisting with any other individual problem presented by relatives in consequence of death.
- Undertaking general liaison duties.

We intend this list to be illustrative rather than prescriptive. There must be recognised training courses for bereavement advisers. Qualification should be certificated, perhaps at a National Vocational Qualification level. Annual assessment and appraisal should be routine and the role should be performance managed. Continuing education and training is essential. The bereavement adviser should work closely with the hospital management, clinicians, the Coroner and the full range of non-medical services including counsellors and other non-medical professionals. There will of course be relatives who do not wish to avail themselves of the services of a bereavement adviser. Nevertheless the service should be offered to everyone as should the facility to return to the bereavement adviser in the event of their services having been declined in the first instance. The distinction between a cardiac liaison nurse and the bereavement adviser is that the nurse has the advantage of contact with the parents in the period prior to death. We suggest that some aspect of the bereavement adviser‘s multi-factorial function will bring them into contact with the parents before the death of their child. We have been heartened at the support for the concept of bereavement adviser from parents and clinicians. We commend the concept for development and implementation.

OPERATIONAL APPROACHES FOR EVALUATING INTERVENTION STRATEGIES

The World Health Organisation (WHO) defines voluntary HIV counselling and testing (VCT) as a confidential dialogue between a client and a care provider aimed at enabling the client to cope with stress and take personal decisions related to HIV/AIDS. Although the effectiveness of this intervention in changing people's behaviour to reduce the risk for HIV infection had been under debate until recently, VCT is already a major component of HIV prevention and care programmes of most developed countries and is being promoted in many developing countries.

The existing literature on counselling and testing is almost exclusively composed of reports on studies that have tried to assess the effects of VCT on behaviour, with before and after intervention evaluation as the most commonly used study design. Very little in the literature addresses issues such as how well the service is provided, how the service is perceived both by the clients and providers, or how cost-effective the service is as provided. This scarcity of information is unfortunate because people affected by HIV/AIDS want HIV counselling and testing services for future planning (including planning for marriage and children), emotional support, medical services, and other referral services4. As such, VCT services require continued, comprehensive (when possible) evaluation to help adapt the service in response to evolving knowledge, client needs, and technology.

This study provides general guidelines for evaluating counselling and testing programmes. Although the goals and objectives of counselling and testing programmes may vary from one country to another and from one programme to another, this study is intended to serve as a practical reference for service providers, programme managers, and those called upon to evaluate HIV prevention programmes.

Evaluating Service Delivery and Service Use

Depending on the goals and objectives of the programme and the interests of the programme managers, an evaluation of service proficiency may cover all aspects related to providing the service or it may focus on one or more specific aspects. The sources of data will also be a function of the aspect of the service to be evaluated. For example, client interviews are an appropriate means to measure clients' satisfaction with the service. Key aspects of VCT services that should be evaluated include counselling and testing protocol adequacy, staff performance, and service accessibility and barriers. Each is discussed below.

Counselling Protocol Adequacy

Counselling and testing protocols may vary from one programme to another based on the goals and objectives of the programme. However, whatever the approach taken, the VCT intervention must be regularly evaluated to determine whether it is provided in accordance with the pre-determined protocol and whether it satisfies clients needs. Results can be used to improve the quality of the service provided. Counselling adequacy is defined by the main components and characteristics of voluntary HIV counselling shown this study.. Questions that must be answered include:

— How well do the counsellors follow the counselling protocol?
— Do the clients feel their confidentiality is protected?
— Is risk assessment conducted? If so, how well is it done?
— Is information provided on HIV transmission and risk factors?
— Is a risk reduction plan discussed?
— Is the meaning of the HIV test explained?
— Is the HIV test result clearly given?
— Is emotional support provided?
— Are referrals for medical and social support provided?
— What is the waiting time at the VCT site?
— Is partner notification conducted? If so, how is it done?

An analysis of the answers to these questions will provide feedback to be used in improving the quality of the service provided.

Objectives of VCT Evaluation

In general, voluntary counselling and testing pursues two interdependent objectives:

— to enable clients to plan and to cope with issues related to HIV/AIDS; and
— to facilitate preventive behaviour

As stated above, the specific objectives of counselling and testing may vary based on the needs expressed or identified during the planning of HIV/AIDS prevention and care programmes. For example, in the United States, HIV counselling and testing is used for surveillance, promoting behaviour change, public education, and referring individuals into treatment and care systems. In most developing countries, counselling and testing programmes are essentially designed to influence clients' risk behaviour and facilitate social and medical support for clients who test positive.

For an evaluation to produce results that will inform the design, implementation, and improvement of VCT programmes, one must take into account the program's objectives. However, whatever the programme objectives are, evaluation activities should address two main areas most relevant for service providers and policymakers:

— Service delivery-How well voluntary counselling and testing is provided

— Programme effectiveness-The intermediate outcomes and long-term impact that voluntary counselling and testing may have on the population receiving the service

Once programme goals and objectives have been clearly defined, the next critical step is selecting appropriate indicators to monitor and evaluate the VCT intervention. Rxamples of programme indicators that may be useful in addressing the different levels of evaluation for voluntary counselling and testing services: service delivery/programme outputs, intermediate programme outcomes, and expected programme impact.

Staff Performance

VCT service requires well-trained and motivated personnel. Regular monitoring of their performance is essential to ensure quality and may help to prevent staff burnout. Focus must be placed on such questions as:

— How well trained are the counsellors?
— How well do counsellors deliver the protocol?
— Are counsellors well informed about other issues relevant to VCT services, including testing technology, options for HIV-positive women who are pregnant, and possible referrals to care and support services?
— How well do counsellors meet clients' needs?
— Are counsellors appropriately supervised?
— Are the counsellors appropriately used?
— What mechanisms are in place to help counsellors solve problems and deal with stress?

Testing Protocol Adequacy

The testing protocol for a VCT service must be designed to reach maximum reliability and validity in accordance with local conditions, such as the type of equipment available, local HIV seroprevalence, and the resources available to acquire the recommended test kits. The testing protocols used in VCT programmes must be examined against the testing strategies for HIV diagnosis recommended by UNAIDS and the World Health Organisation to ensure that they are adequate for the local context. The evaluation of the testing protocol must provide answers to the following questions:

— How consistently is the protocol used?
— How valid is the testing algorithm in terms of specificity and sensitivity?
— How long must clients wait to receive their test result? Are clients comfortable with the waiting period?
— How much does the testing protocol cost?

— Is the testing protocol the most appropriate given local conditions? If not, how can it be improved?

Service Use

The extent to which services are used is an important factor in determining the viability of a programme. A VCT service with a minimal level of use by the target population is not cost-effective and therefore unlikely to receive support and continued funding, even if it is effective in other ways. An evaluation of service use must answer the following questions:

— Who uses the service?

— How many clients are served?

— Why do people seek the service?

— Do clients complete all procedures involved in using the service?

— Is the level of use sufficient to justify sustaining the service?

Service Accessibility and Barriers

It is important to identify factors that affect accessibility and create potential barriers to service use. Parameters to be evaluated include:

— How far must the intended population travel to reach the service?

— Is public transportation to the VCT site available?

— How much does it cost for clients to receive VCT services?

Because clients must pay for medical services in many developing countries, it is essential that cost does not become a barrier to individuals using the service, especially those who might need it the most. When assessing accessibility, it is also important for those who are planning an evaluation to keep in mind that being near to a VCT site does not always guarantee easy access to the service. In fact, in areas where there are strong stigmas attached to HIV/ AIDS, proximity can be a barrier to service use because potential clients may prefer to go to a VCT site far away from the sight of their neighbors, who may suspect them of being infected just because they visited a VCT center. In this context, it is also important to assess who is being reached by the VCT site:

— Are those at highest risk obtaining the services?

— Are significant populations or groups not being reached?

Sources of Data

Evaluation data on VCT service delivery and use can be obtained from various sources. Service records and the staff of counselling and testing sites are an important source of information for the evaluation of VCT services. The sites' records may be used to collect data on the level of service use, the characteristics of clients attending the sites, reasons for using counselling and testing service, and the testing protocol being used. Standard forms containing relevant information must be developed and filled out on a regular basis by the VCT staff. These can be used later for evaluation purposes. The staff of VCT sites may provide useful information about their perception of the quality of the service provided to clients, possible barriers to service use by potential clients, the level and quality of supervision provided to counsellors, but also information on the impact-physical, emotional, and otherwise-that counselling and testing has on its providers. Information on these issues may be obtained through periodic key informant interviews or focus group discussions, if appropriate.

Clients can provide information on all aspects of VCT service delivery and use. These data may be obtained through exit interviews with a subsample of randomly selected consenting clients after a counselling session using a standardized questionnaire that focuses on the clients' perceptions of the quality of the session and the counsellor's performance, or their impressions of the VCT site in general (for example, accessibility of the site, perceived barriers to use, organisation of the service, ability of the service to meet client needs, length of waiting time, cost of the service). In-depth interviews and focus group discussions with a selected number of clients may be used to collect additional contextual information. Non-participant observers as well as "professional customers" (or mystery clients) may be used to conduct quality assurance activities through direct observation of the VCT procedures. Direct observation can help in assessing the adequacy of counselling and testing protocols and the adequacy of the counselling and testing actually provided (staff performance). Some practical issues related to direct observation must be addressed before it is used, however. For example, clients may be concerned about the confidentiality of the information they reveal if there is a third person in the room during the counselling session. The presence of an observer may also alter the natural way a counsellor interacts with his/her client. Efforts must be made to reassure clients and minimize pressure on the staff being monitored.

Surveys of the population at large, which include former, current, and potential VCT service users, or surveys of selected populations, such as hard-to-reach groups in defined catchment areas of the site, provide complementary information about the performance of the VCT service as perceived by the community. In addition, population-based surveys may help to identify what the population expects from the service as well as barriers to service use. Such surveys will also provide information that can be used to characterize people who use and do not use the service, and identify ways to improve the service and make it more accessible and attractive to the population.

Randomised Design

A randomized controlled design-by far the most rigorous way to measure VCT effectiveness-may be used so long as it is assured that participants in the control group also receive a beneficial intervention. Different VCT protocols may be tested using this design. For example, same-day testing may be compared to the standard protocol requiring the client to return in a week or two for the test results. Or, a two-session counselling protocol (pre- and post-test counselling) may be compared to an open protocol in which a client uses as much counselling as needed. Counselling and testing programmes may also be compared with other prevention interventions. Given the high cost of this experimental design and the scarce resources in most developing countries, programme managers must carefully weigh the relevance of this design before embarking on a randomized controlled intervention. It should be used only when there is an important conceptual question to be answered that will have regional or international significance. In reality, few programmes will ever conduct such trials because of their expense and methodologic complexity.

Pre-Post Intervention Client Surveys

With this approach, a random sample of clients seen at the VCT site(s) is selected to be followed for a given time period. A standardized behavioural survey questionnaire is administered to the selected clients before they receive any intervention and the same questionnaire is administered to them some time (1, 3, or 6 months) after the intervention.

To enhance this evaluation approach, data on STI status should be collected from the clients at intake and follow-up to support the survey findings. Although less expensive and complex than a randomized controlled trial design, such surveys are not easy to conduct in resource poor settings and the results are often considerably biased due to substantial follow-up losses. Moreover, a pre-post intervention design with no comparison group does not allow evaluators to control for behaviour-modifying effects that are unrelated to expected intervention effects.

Nevertheless, the evaluation of the AIDS Information Center in Kampala, Uganda, is an example of this approach. Another example is the work by Kamenga and colleagues in Kinshasa, Congo (former Zaire), where married couples were interviewed on sexual behaviour before receiving voluntary HIV counselling and testing. Discordant couples (one partner HIV-positive and the other HIV-negative) were then followed and assessed monthly for behaviour change (questionnaire) and STI incidence (laboratory testing). There is now increasing support for expanded programmes of voluntary counselling and testing to enable people to cope with issues related to HIV/AIDS, to encourage preventive behaviours, and to facilitate access to care and support services for people who test positive for HIV. To ensure continued quality and inform programmatic improvement, evaluating VCT services must be an ongoing process that is integrated into the implementation of the service from the beginning. Evaluative activities will be determined on the basis of programme objectives and the available funds for evaluation.

For practical and operational purposes, the evaluation of VCT interventions should focus on key service aspects, such as service use, the adequacy of counselling and testing protocols, staff performance, and service accessibility, and should use complementary sources of information that provide different perspectives on the various service performance aspects. These sources include VCT staff and service records, client surveys, direct observation of VCT service provision, and population surveys in the community reached by the programme. Special emphasis must be given to ensuring the confidentiality of sensitive information revealed by clients or VCT staff. The data collected must be analysed and used to ultimately provide feedback to all interested parties at different levels (from the staff to the central authorities) and the methodology used must be carefully selected taking in account programme priorities and available resources.

Programme outcomes related to behaviour change, stigma reduction, and community support should be assessed periodically to determine the extent to which voluntary counselling and testing services have achieved their intermediate programme goals and objectives. Measures of the long-term programme impact should include trends in mother-to-child transmission of HIV in women of childbearing age because voluntary counselling and testing services play an essential role in interventions designed to reduce this mode of HIV transmission.

Evaluating Outcomes And Impact (Effectiveness) Of VCT Programmes

Effectiveness evaluation of VCT programmes aims to determine how well voluntary counselling and testing services have achieved their intermediate and long-term programme goals. Intermediate outcome indicators may measure the extent to which the VCT intervention has encouraged behaviour change among clients and their partners and changes in STI rates as a biological proxy indicator for adopting preventive behaviours. Other important outcome indicators should measure the reduction in stigma of, and discrimination against, HIV/AIDS-affected people in the community. Measures of long-term programme impact attempt to determine whether VCT intervention activities have affected the rate of HIV transmission in the community, including mother-to-child transmission. They should also include an assessment of the impact of VCT on societal norms in the community reached by the programme. To approach this difficult task and be able to make meaningful inferences on programme effectiveness, evaluators must analyse VCT process data together with other types of data that are collected in the catchment area of VCT services. These data include behavioural survey data, HIV sentinel data, and ethnographic research data.

A recent multicenter randomized trial conducted by the AIDSCAP Project of Family Health International and UNAIDS/WHO in three developing countries has demonstrated the effectiveness of VCT in changing sexual behaviour of those counseled and tested. However, although VCT has demonstrated its effectiveness in changing risk behaviour in these selected study sites, VCT programme managers still must determine whether the VCT service they provide makes a difference for those who receive it. An effective counselling model in one community may not be as effective in another community. Different models may have to be tried to identify the most effective one for a given setting. The following descriptions of different outcome and impact evaluation approaches show how the effectiveness of particular VCT services can be assessed.

UNDERSTANDING THIRD-PARTY CARRIERS: TIPS FOR RHEUMATOLOGISTS AND THEIR STAFFS

Since almost all of a rheumatologist's income comes from third-party reimbursement, it is important to understand how the health insurance reimbursement process works. A brief guide is included in this study, although you are encouraged to do further research regarding carriers in your area.

Commercial Carriers

Commercial carriers are private, for-profit companies that provide group and/or individual plans. Premiums and coverage are determined by each company (e.g., Aetna, Prudential and Travelers). Commercial carriers have historically offered traditional indemnity health plans that reimburse fee-for-service with the insurance covering 80 percent of the health plan allowance and the patient being held responsible for the remaining 20 percent copayment. Most commercial insurance plans have predefined patient deductibles and copayment provisions. Generally, physicians do not have special contract agreements with commercial carriers.

Types of Third-Party Payors

There are several major types of third-party payors: commercial carriers; Blue Cross/Blue Shield plans; government programmes such as Medicare, Medicaid, CHAMPUS/CHAMPVA and Worker's Compensation; as well as alternate health plans such as health maintenance organisations, preferred provider organisations, point-of-service plans and self-funded plans.

Health Maintenance Organisations (HMOs)

HMOs provide comprehensive health care ranging from physician services to hospitalisation. Patients enrolled in HMOs are entitled to the full range of services offered by the HMO with their payment of a fixed amount per month (or other payment period) during their period of enrollment. In addition to their fixed monthly enrollment payments, the patient is usually responsible for a small copayment for visits to the physician, and the patient has a selected group of physicians from which he or she may seek care.

There are four different HMO models:

— *Staff Model HMOs* employ physicians who are typically paid a salary to provide services to HMO patients
— *Group Model HMOs* primarily contract with larger, multispecialty physician groups. The physicians are employees of the group practice, not the HMO (in order to gain access to HMO patients, a physician must be a member of a group practice which contracts with the HMO)
— *Independent Practice Association (IPA) Model HMOs* are entities which have one or more managed care contracts, and in turn contract with independent physician groups for all specialties to provide the services to fulfill those contracts (the HMO pays a capitation fee to the IPA and in turn, the IPA pays the member physicians, usually on a fee-for-service basis, as services are rendered to the HMO patients)
— *Network or Direct-Contract Model HMOs* contract with physicians at all levels and usually use a combination of each model type (physician reimbursement may vary between capitation and discounted fee-for-service)

Blue Cross/Blue Shield Plans

Blue Cross/Blue Shield plans are a federation of individual, usually not-for-profit plans which typically operate only in the state in which they are located. These plans contract directly with physician, hospitals and various other health entities to provide services to their insured companies and individuals. Blue Cross plans primarily provide hospital services, outpatient care, some institutional services and home care. Blue Shield provides physician services (and in some cases dental, outpatient and vision care). Most BC/BS plans offer health maintenance organisations, preferred provider organisations and point-of-service plans in addition to group and individual fee-for-service plans.

In some areas, participation in a Blue Shield plan is renewed on a yearly basis. Be sure you receive a copy of the contract and understand it before you sign it.

Medicare: This is a federal health insurance programme for individuals aged 65 or older, people of any age with permanent kidney failure or end-stage renal disease, and certain disabled people. It is administered by the Health Care Financing Administration (HCFA).

Part A of Medicare provides hospital insurance benefits for the aged, disabled and blind for inpatient and certain follow-up care. These benefits are provided to enrollees by the federal government. *Part B* of Medicare provides medical insurance which pays for doctors' services and supplies not covered by Part A. A monthly premium, which is set annually by the federal government, is paid by enrollees.

Medicaid: This is a health insurance plan sponsored by both the federal and state governments. Coverage is administered on a state-specific basis, although general federal guidelines are followed. Medicaid is an assistance programme available in all states in various forms. Physicians enroll as providers with the Department of Public Health or the Department of Human Services in their states. Worker's Compensation: This is a state required insurance programme in which employers are responsible for premiums and maintenance. The risk involved in the employee's job determines the amount of insurance to be carried. Worker's Compensation laws are state-specific and vary regarding reporting coverage and benefit waiting periods.

CHAMPUS/CHAMPVA (Civilian Health and Medical

Programme of the Uniformed Services/ Veterans Administration): This programme provides comprehensive health benefits for families of uniformed services personnel and service retirees as a supplement to military and Public Health Service care. This programme is federally funded and is administered by the Office for the Civilian Health and Medical Programme of the Uniformed Services (OCHAMPUS).

Preferred Provider Organisations (PPOs)

Generally, a PPO is a group of health care providers including physicians, hospitals and allied institutions that agree to provide services to a specific pool of patients. PPOs have been offered by insurance carriers, groups of physicians and groups of hospitals. Under PPOs, the physician's reimbursement is based on a discounted fee schedule, and payment is based on traditional fee-for-service billing. Because each PPO plan varies in coverage and benefit packages, practices should review each PPO contract presented to them and be aware of the plan's discounted fee schedule, contract requirements and potential risk. Furthermore, policies and procedures for claim submission vary as well.

What Happens When You Submit a Claim?

When you mail the claim form to the carrier, it is date-stamped upon receipt. Much of the information encoded or written on the form is entered into the carrier's computerized claims processing system by data entry personnel. If you transmit your claims electronically, this step is omitted. In either instance, the claim is subjected to an automated review to determine if deductibles have been met, if the services for which the claim has been submitted are covered, and if your charge for the service is "reasonable." In addition, this review will also begin to determine the medical necessity of the services provided; therefore, the diagnosis must relate to the procedures you perform. "Utilisation screens" are built into the computer's review process. These are predetermined frequency parameters for specific types of services that sift out claims for further review. Claims that are "screened" out for manual review are then examined by a claims reviewer (an employee of the carrier who is trained to review and process medical claims but who may have no medical training), a nurse or a physician. At this point, pre-established carrier medical policies are applied to claim situations. These policies are developed by medical professionals, usually physicians, in consultation with the carrier. Medical specialists or societies may also be involved in the Medicare programme — many Medicare carriers use physicians on their Carrier Advisory Committees. Claims reviewers are required to review all of the information on the form and any supporting documentation that has been submitted.

Self-funded Plans

Self-funded plans are instituted by large corporations, frequently managed by a third-party administrator. The third party administrator establishes a PPO or similar type of arrangement with physicians, hospitals, and other health care providers. To institute a self-funded plan, the corporation must obtain an excess liability rider and establish a reserve fund to pay employee medical bills. The remainder of this study generally describes the claims submission process, as well as strategies that you can use to take control of the process. In most cases, these strategies apply to claims submitted to any carrier. Some of the information presented is specific to the Medicare carrier review process. In such instances, Medicare has been referenced specifically.

6 Steps to Filing Insurance Claims Successfully

The following steps to completing insurance claims forms

should help to increase the likelihood that you will be reimbursed for the services you provide your patients. You are also encouraged to refer to manuals prepared by your own carriers for additional specific information.

Step 1: Billing Identification Numbers. Include the appropriate billing identification numbers on the insurance claim forms.

Step 2: Code Correctly. Miscoded claims or use of the wrong claim forms are guaranteed to cause reimbursement delays and frustration. These claims require manual review because they are not written in the "languages" your carriers' computers understand, CPT and ICD-9-CM. You must learn to "speak" these languages if you want your carrier to understand what you did and to reimburse you for it. Claims reviewers are rarely rheumatologists. Relying on them to select the appropriate codes for what they think you did is risky. This may result in a lower reimbursement for you or your patients. Order CPT and ICD-9-CM books yearly so you will have all the updated information. Furthermore, you put yourself at risk if you expect your staff to code correctly for services you performed, especially if your patient reports consist of symbols, acronyms or abbreviations not listed in the coding index. Help your staff help you by participating in the coding process. It will also be to your advantage to code legibly. If the claims reviewer cannot decipher your handwriting, your office may be contacted by telephone or in writing for an explanation or clarification. This will slow down the reimbursement process. The reviewer may, however, take a guess as to what you reported. This may result in a lower reimbursement or even a denial. Claims that are legible, preferably typewritten (or in a dark blue or black ink when handwritten) can be processed more quickly and accurately. If your claim form is not completed in full, it will be suspended for manual review.

All forms should be double-checked by your billing staff to be sure that all of the necessary information has been correctly included. If you ask your Medicare patient to sign an advance notice agreeing to pay for the services you provided, you should enclose a copy of the notice for the Medicare carrier. Be sure to keep a copy in the patient's chart as well. A notice given out on a routine basis which does no more than state that Medicare payment denial is possible is not an acceptable advance notice. It must be individualized for the service on a specific date. A sample advance notice is included in the appendix of this manual.

Step 3: Use ICD-9-CM Codes. All carriers require information regarding the diagnosis, so you must include the appropriate ICD-9-CM code. This information is cross-matched to the service or procedure by the carrier to justify what was done. Remember, each service or procedure (CPT code) must relate specifically to a particular diagnosis (ICD-9-CM code). Also, the ICD-9-CM code should be coded to the highest level of specificity, or fifth digit. A match determined to be inappropriate by the carrier may result in a request for further clarification, once again resulting in slower payment. Worse still, the claim may simply be denied. Codes are added and deleted yearly in the ICD-9-CM code book.

Step 4: Document, Document, Document. It helps to anticipate what the reviewer will need in order to process the claims. Provide additional documentation to support your claim. Call the reviewer's attention to this supplementary documentation by noting it on the claim form. Then staple it to the form. Every service submitted for payment must be documented in the patient's records. This includes diagnostic tests, medical care, surgery and any other services eligible for payment. If you see a patient in the hospital, document the visit and date, and note the medical necessity supporting the reason for your visit in the hospital record and on the claim form. This can help to confirm that the visit actually occurred and it may help to justify the need for the visit if it is questioned.

Step 5: Communicate With Carriers in Writing. It is always better to communicate with your carrier in writing rather than by telephone. This allows you to maintain an accurate record of what you requested, the person(s) you contacted, and the response you received. Should you find yourself in an appeal situation, such a record may be extremely useful.

Step 6: Reconsideration. If you do not agree with the reimbursement of a procedure, you may ask for reconsideration of your claim. Send an explanation of why you do not agree along with supportive documentation to the carrier.

Overpayment Notices

If you receive a refund notice from Medicare questioning the medical necessity of a service or procedure you provided, the following checklist might help you to resolve the problem:

(a) Have you included all the necessary basic information on the claim form and attached supporting documentation to it?

(b) Are the codes and other descriptive information you included about the service or procedure accurate?

(c) Would the carrier automatically know that the CPT and ICD-9-CM codes you used "match"?

(d) If you can answer "no" to any of the above, have you explained the inconsistencies?

If you still don't know why the carrier is questioning the medical necessity of your claim, ask the carrier! In the case of Medicare, HCFA has instructed carriers to provide a "clear carrier point of contact" with each medically unnecessary notice they send. Other insurers may not be as helpful. In any case, when you have unanswered questions, call or write the carrier and ask for a clarification about missing information or what else may be required to help the carrier understand the medical necessity of what you did. If you call, remember to document the conversation and the information you received.

There is a list of Medicare carriers by state in the appendix of this manual. If you have any questions about Medicare policy regarding medical necessity determinations, write for clarification. At this point, either the Medicare carrier will agree that the services you provided were medically necessary and your claim will be paid, or you will receive a denial notice from the carrier. Such notices include the reason(s) the carrier believes the services were not medically necessary, as well as refund regulations. From Medicare's perspective, you can either issue a refund to your patient or credit his or her account. You also have a right to appeal the refund decision.

How to Avoid Medical Necessity Reductions

You can avoid medical necessity reductions by classifying patient visits accurately to reflect the level of E/M service you actually provided. Do not get into the habit of coding patient visits or consultations in a "routine" fashion. All patient visits should be coded on an individual basis and not classified in particular categories. Carriers' computer programmes are designed to track coding patterns. If, for example, all of your claims for patients with osteoarthritis are coded at the same level of E/M service, your carrier may request a justification from you to support the medical necessity of that level of care for such claims.

PROCEDURES FOR OBTAINING INFORMED CONSENT

The process of obtaining informed consent, whether a written document or an oral communication, is one means of ensuring that patients understand the risks and benefits of a treatment or medical intervention. Rooted in medical ethics and codified as a legal principle, it is based on the assertion that a competent individual has the right to determine what will or will not be done to him or her. The American Medical Association (AMA) Code of Medical Ethics establishes informed consent as an ethical obligation of physicians. In addition to being an ethical obligation of physicians, legislation in all 50 states requires that patients be informed of all important aspects of a treatment and/or procedures, although the details of these laws and statutes differ greatly. Failure to obtain adequate informed consent renders a physician liable for negligence or battery and constitutes medical malpractice.

To date, studies of informed consent have not investigated outcomes related to the adequacy of the communication, insofar as this may impact patient safety. Physician-patient communication styles have been linked to lower rates of malpractice claims. Nonetheless, as noted by Levinson, malpractice claims do not reflect the actual rate of negligence. While some have hypothesized that better informed consent could improve the patient-physician relationship, establish trust, increase patient compliance, and provide information that could reduce medical error, this has not been shown. In the absence of a direct link between adequate informed consent and the reduction of medical error, the "patient safety outcome" reviewed in this study is the patient's provision of adequate informed consent.

Prevalence and Severity of Target Safety Problem

Procedures to obtain consent must ensure that the

patient understands his or her condition, as well as the risk and benefits of treatment, and its alternatives. It has been estimated that less than half of the US population understands commonly used medical terms. This "health literacy" problem may impact the ability of the patient to understand any attempts to obtain information. In addition to lack of comprehension, procedures to obtain informed consent may be incomplete.

Several studies have noted the various insufficiencies in procedures to obtain informed consent. Three studies examined the completeness of physician-patient conversations in obtaining informed consent. Braddock et al focused on outpatient discussions. Recognizing that some procedures may require more discussion than others, they created a three-tiered evaluation procedure, in which the completeness of patient-physician discussions differ according to the complexity of the decision being discussed.

Basic decisions, such as laboratory tests, require the least in-depth discussion, covering only the patient's role, the clinical nature of the decision, and exploration of patient preferences. Intermediate decisions, such as changes in medication, require a moderate depth of discussion, incorporating the Tier 1 subjects, and adding a discussion of alternative treatments, the risks and benefits of the alternatives, and an assessment of the patients understanding.

Complex decisions such as surgery require a discussion of the uncertainties associated with the decision, in addition to all of the aforementioned steps. Analysing audiotaped conversations between 1057 patients and 59 primary-care physicians and 65 surgeons, Braddock et al found that 17.2% of basic decisions contained all required components, while none of the intermediate decisions and only one of the complex decisions contained all of the required components. Applying only the Tier 1 basic consent standards, 20.5% of basic decisions, 21.9% of intermediate decisions, and 38.2% of complex decisions met all the criteria.

In a study of informed consents of surrogates for pediatric patients undergoing surgery, coders examined audiotaped conversations with surrogates, as well as structured interview and questionnaire data regarding the conversations. They noted that patients' recall of the conversations with physicians often omitted key components, such as the risks and benefits of the procedures.

Bottrell et al examined the completeness of 540 consent forms from 157 hospitals nationwide. Of these, 26.4% included all four of the basic elements (risks, benefits, alternatives, and other important aspects of the procedure). Eighty-seven percent noted the general possibility of risk, but less than half provided specific information. Alternatives were noted in 56.9% of the forms, and benefits appeared in 37%, though most of these were general references rather than specific information. Although 74% of consent forms were deemed incomplete, it is unknown whether physician-patient discussions that preceded the signing of the consent form included the missing information.

A study by Mark et al found that 82.4% of 102 participants reported that they understood everything that their physicians had described about a procedure and indicated that all of their questions had been answered. Eighteen patients had remaining unanswered questions. Half of this group requested more time to speak with their physicians, while the other 9 felt that their questions were not important.

In a study by Lavelle-Jones, 69% of patients admitted that they did not read a consent form before signing it. In addition, approximately half of the patients awaiting treatment were unhappy with the amount of information they received, with 21% stating that most of the information they obtained about their surgical treatment was obtained outside of the hospital.

Consent forms have been targeted for their lack of readability. Patients with limited reading ability are at increased risk for medical errors, due to problems reading medication bottles, appointment slips, self-care instructions, and health education brochures. These patients may also have trouble reading materials intended to aid in obtaining informed consent. According to the National Adult Literacy Survey of 1993, approximately 40-44 million Americans were functionally illiterate, defined as the inability to complete basic reading tasks required to function as a member of society. In addition, even in educated adults, the highest grade-level completed may not reflect actual reading comprehension level. A study of 100 adult cancer patients found that most read at a mean grade-level equivalent of between 10 and 11 grade. The authors suggest that forms and educational materials be written at a grade-level three levels below the highest level of education completed by a patient.

Several studies have examined the readability of procedure consent forms. Two studies examined consent forms for radiologic procedures using computer generated "readability" scores. Consent forms for use with iodinated contrast media found that 12.35 years of education were required to read consent forms. A similar study of general radiologic procedure consent forms found that they required a mean of 15 years of education. Only 16% of forms could be understood by patients with a high-school education. Another Hopper et al study found that general hospital consent forms were written at a grade level of 12.6. Just over half could be understood by a patient with a high school education, less than a third by patients with a 10 grade reading level, and just over 5% by patients with an 8 grade reading level.

Practice Description

Informed consent is a process through which a physician informs a patient about the risks and benefits of a proposed therapy and allows the patient to decide whether the therapy will be undertaken. It may be received in one sitting, or over a period of time, either orally or in writing or a combination of the two. Informed consent procedures have been instituted in both research and clinical medicine. In the former case, federal regulations establish strict guidelines for informed consent that are monitored by a special board at each institution (Institutional Review Board). In addition, risks and adverse events that occur while research is in progress are followed closely and reported. As such, informed consent in the research setting differs greatly from informed consent in the clinical setting. In clinical practice, formal efforts, such as the signing of a consent form, (presumably preceded by adequate exchange of information), are only undertaken in some circumstances, notably prior to major invasive procedures such as radiologic procedures and surgery. Less well appreciated is that all medical care, including pharmacy prescriptions or laboratory tests, requires informal informed consent, except when the patient is incompetent to make a decision or relinquishes the right to provide it. Studies suggest that in practice only minimal formal efforts are made to obtain informed consent for routine interventions.

Legislation governing the requirements of, and conditions under which, consent must be obtained varies greatly from State to State. General guidelines, such as those proposed by the AMA require patients to be informed of the nature of their condition and the proposed procedure, the purpose of the procedure, the risks and benefits of the proposed treatments, the probability of the anticipated risks and benefits, alternatives to the treatment and the associated risks and benefits, and the risks and benefits of not receiving the treatment or procedure.

As discussed below, procedures to obtain informed consent may not adequately promote the patient's comprehension of the information provided, rendering the consent not truly "informed." Interventions that may prove beneficial in improving and ensuring the patient's understanding include redrafting of consent forms to reduce complexity, providing written materials to accompany oral conversations, using multimedia or other techniques to improve comprehension, and asking patients to recap discussions about the procedure.

Opportunities for Impact

While informed consent is a well-established practice, it often fails to meet its stated purpose. Several methods of improving the procedures of obtaining informed consent have been proposed, including improving the readability of consent forms, asking patients for recall to establish understanding, adding additional stimuli, such as multimedia presentations and providing written information.

Lavelle-Jones found that elderly patients (over 60 years of age) had poorer recall than younger patients. In addition, patients with internal locus of control—those who believed their health was in their own control—were better informed than those with an external locus of control. Patients with above average IQ exhibited better recall. These findings could indicate "at-risk" groups that interventions may target.

One author argues that an important opportunity for impact is to change the model of implementing informed consent from a single event approach to a process approach. Currently obtaining informed consent often revolves around the signing of the consent form. Although this approach clearly delineates the responsibility of healthcare providers, provides documentation of the consent, and fits easily into the current provider structure, it often results in patients failing to actually comprehend the information and reinforces physicians' conception that the consent ritual is futile. In contrast, a process model involves the physician providing information over time, establishing a better patient-physician relationship and better comprehension of medical care. As of yet there is no data to support these suppositions.

Since the definition of adequate informed consent is debatable, the number of individuals currently not receiving interventions to obtain adequate informed consent is likely to be quite high, but is not known.

Study Design, Outcomes and Effectiveness of Various Approaches

Structured Discussions

Informed consent is often obtained during informal discussion between physicians or nurses and patients, and (as discussed above), these discussions frequently do not cover all of the relevant information. Two studies examined the use of a structured interview format in providing information to patients. Solomon et al studied 36 patients receiving cardiac catheterisation for the first time at a Veterans hospital. Patients were randomized into two groups (Level 1 design). Both groups were briefed by a cardiologist regarding the procedure (standard care). In addition, the experimental group received a 30-minute structured teaching session with a nurse to discuss all aspects of the procedure, including the purposes, techniques, sensations, risks and benefits. Patients in the experimental group also received an illustrated guide to cardiovascular procedures and an educational pamphlet. All subjects were tested using a 13-item questionnaire covering the information that should have been imparted during informed consent procedures (Level 3 outcome). The intervention group scored significantly better than the control group.

Improving Readability of Consent Forms and Education Materials

In order to ensure that patients understand the procedure to which they are consenting, it is important that all materials be presented in a comprehensible manner. Consent forms are written with relatively complex sentence structure and vocabulary, making it difficult for the average adult to interpret the information. In addition, providing consent forms in the primary language of patients may improve consent procedures. However, we located no studies examining the effectiveness of such practices. In a later study, Dawes et al studied 190 hospitalized patients undergoing ENT surgery. Patients were assigned to one of 4 groups. Groups 1 and 2 were assigned at different times (Level 2 design), while groups 3 and 4 were randomly assigned (Level 1 design). Group 1 had no consent interview until after assessment at the conclusion of the study. Group 2 engaged in an informal interview with a physician (reflecting current practice), during which the number of complications discussed was recorded. Group 3 engaged in a structured interview with a physician, covering the purpose and technique of the procedure, complications, sensations, alternatives, and benefits (a checklist was used as a guide). The final group, Group 4, engaged in the same structured interview, except that the patient was provided with a copy of the checklist and allowed to take it with them after the interview. Patient anxiety was assessed following consent using a visual analog scale, then reassessed at an interview, given 4 hours later. At the later interview, patients were asked to recount orally the operation name, describe what would be done, list complications, and state whether they understood the information given to them (Level 3 outcome). All but Group 1 (control group) patients showed a drop to normal anxiety after informed consent. Group 2 (informal discussion) remembered proportionately more complications mentioned in the informal interview, although fewer complication were covered. Groups 3 and 4 recalled more total complications than Group 2. There was no differences between Groups 3 and 4 (structured interviews).

Asking for Recall

A simple method of determining whether a patient understands information regarding a procedure is to ask the patient to recount what he or she has been told. Two studies examined this intervention, using a randomized controlled trial design (Level 1 design). In the first study, informed consent was solicited from 50 patients undergoing percutaneous lung biopsy. Twenty-seven patients in the control group were offered the standard procedure for obtaining informed consent: approximately 30 minutes prior to the procedure, the physician described the procedure in detail, including its risks and benefits. Four complications were specifically described, along with their relative risks. Patients were asked to sign a standard consent form. Twenty-three patients received the same procedure, but in addition, they were asked to describe all 4 potential complications. The procedure was repeated until all patients in the intervention group could recount all of the complications. This modified procedure usually took less than 5 minutes extra compared with the traditional approach. Patients were interviewed 2 hours after the procedure was completed. Patients in the modified consent group had better recall (Level 2 outcome) than patients in the control group (56%

vs. 14% with high recall (recalling 3-4 out of 4 risks), and 13% vs. 44% with low recall (recalling 0-1 out of 4 risks)).

A second study examined verbalisation in 20 patients undergoing anterior cruciate ligament (ACL) reconstruction. Patients were randomly assigned to 2 groups. Both groups received the standard education for ACL reconstruction, which included the use of a 3-D model of the knee, discussion with a physician about the procedure, and obtaining informed consent. The experimental group (8 subjects) also were asked to repeat back the risks of the procedure until they could accurately recall all risks discussed. One-month later, recall regarding the information received was tested using a 3-item questionnaire (Level 2 outcome). All 8 in the experimental group answered all questions correctly, while only four out of the 12 in the control group answered all questions correctly (p=0.03).

Use of Visual or Auditory Learning Aids

Adding additional stimuli may increase the ability of the patient to understand information being conveyed or increase retention of that information. For instance, use of visual diagrams may make a procedure easier to understand. Multi-media may also promote better comprehension. Three studies have examined the addition of visual stimuli for informed consent. One study of patients undergoing back surgery examined the impact of a diagnosis-specific videodisk programme on patient outcomes. Patients (n=393) who were candidates for elective back surgery (primarily for herniated disc and spinal stenosis) were randomized to two education groups (Level 1 design). The control group received a written booklet regarding the surgical and non-surgical treatments for herniated disc and spinal stenosis, a description of expected outcomes, and a short self-test on the booklet information. Patients in the experimental group also received the booklet, but in addition viewed a videodisk programme. The programme allowed a patient to enter their diagnosis and age and receive customized information on the alternative treatments, discussion of the diagnoses (and the ambiguities of diagnosis), and interviews from patients that had been treated surgically and non-surgically. At the end the patient was provided with a printout of outcome probabilities. Patients in the experimental group were slightly more likely to report that they had all the information they wanted (Level 3 outcome). Rates of patients consenting to surgery for herniated disk (32% vs. 47%) and other diagnoses (5.4% vs. 14.0%) were lower in the videodisk group.

Hopper et al also tested an interactive video programme, although the tested programme was computer based. One-hundred and sixty outpatients referred for IV contrast media studies were stratified by age, sex, and previous exposure to contrast media, then randomized to receive either a written consent form, or an interactive computer-based video (Level 1 design). Subjects in the control group received a consent form designed to be read at an eighth grade reading level. Subjects in the experimental group viewed a video in which a physician used identical words as the consent form to inform subjects about the procedure and risks. Subjects then had an option of hearing more about the risks. If subjects chose not to hear additional information, they were provided with printouts of the risks (with the minimal information already given). Otherwise, subjects were provided with printouts certifying that they had completed the programme. All subjects were tested using a 7-item questionnaire regarding the procedure and risks (Level 2 outcome). Patients that viewed the video responded correctly more often than the control group when asked about general aspects of the procedure. Female patients in the video group also responded correctly more often to questions about risks, although this finding did not hold for male patients. The video did take approximately 1.6 minutes of additional time to complete, and there was no difference in patients desire for additional knowledge between the groups (Level 3 outcome).

One final study did not use an interactive video, but tested whether providing information via video was superior to providing information via an informal discussion with the physician (standard practice). Two-hundred and twenty four subjects referred for colonoscopy were stratified into previous or no previous colonoscopy, then randomized into 3 groups (Level 1 design). The control group had a structured discussion with a physician, in which the physician covered the same information covered in the video according to a checklist. The video-only group watched a 5-minute videotape, in which a physician described the procedure, and its risk and benefits. The third group (video and discussion), watched the video and then engaged in a structured discussion with a physician. All patients were tested using a 13-item questionnaire (Level 2 outcome). Both video groups gave more correct responses than the discussion-only group, although they did not differ from each other. In addition, patient anxiety levels were measured using the State-Trait Anxiety Inventory (Level 3 outcome). There were no differences among the 3 groups.

Providing Written Information to Patients

Providing written information to patients regarding their diagnoses, proposed treatments, and other information given during informed consent discussion allows the patient to refer back to such information, and possibly increases comprehension. One early study compared the then-common practice, informal interview between patient and doctor, with provision of a written consent form. Eighty patients, referred for a first excretory urography, were randomly assigned to 2 groups (Level 1 design). The control group received standard care, the informal interview. The experimental group received the same interview along with a detailed written consent form to read and sign. Patient clinical reactions and side effects were monitored (Level 1 outcome). One to 3 days after the procedures, patients retrospectively rated discomfort, fear or apprehension, and understanding of the procedure (Level 3 outcome). Patients also completed an 8-item knowledge examination covering the information on the consent form (Level 2 outcome), or in the informal interview. Experimental subjects scored significantly better (p=<0.01) than control subjects for the knowledge exam (scoring 73% vs. 48%), but did not differ in their discomfort, perception of the procedure, or anxiety.

Some investigators have proposed that patients should receive written consent forms days before receiving a procedure. Neptune et al studied 160 subjects referred for a contrast media radiology exam. The patients were stratified by age, sex, and previous exposure to contrast media, and then were randomized within the strata into 2 groups (Level 1 design). The control group received a simple consent form (designed such that it could be read with an eighth grade education), 15-60 minutes before the procedure, consistent with standard care. Patients in the experimental group received the same consent form 24-72 hours before the procedure, and were called one day in advance to remind them to read the form. Subjects' knowledge concerning their procedures was tested using a 7-item questionnaire (Level 2 outcome). Overall, there were no significant differences between the two groups on either a knowledge or satisfaction score.

In a British study, 265 patients undergoing intrathoracic, intraperitoneal, or vascular procedures, were assigned to one of 2 consent groups (Level 2 design). The control group was provided with an oral explanation of their disease and the proposed procedures. Members in the experimental group were provided with the same information, and also provided with an "operation card" detailing the same information. Patients were given 30 minutes to review the cards before signing the consent form. Patients were interviewed for recall (Level 2 outcome) immediately after consent (1 hour), the day of discharge, 4-6 weeks post-discharge, and at 6 months post-discharge. Control and experimental groups did not differ, except on the day of discharge ($p<0.0001$). The only significant factor in predicting recall was the age of the patient, as older patients had poorer recall than younger patients, even when controlling for psychological factors. Written information did not appear to aid in recall for older patients at any time point.

Two other studies provided written information to patients, although this was combined with structured teaching programmes. These studies are reviewed under "Structured Discussions" above.

Comment

While much has been written regarding informed consent and the ethical obligations of providers to obtain proper informed consent, serious shortcomings have been reported. However, very little literature has examined the impact of different procedures for obtaining informed consent on the quality of the consent obtained. The weight of the literature suggests that the value of informed consent can be modestly enhanced by augmenting standard provider-patient discussions with additional learning and retention aids (written or videodisk materials). Moreover, the process of consent can be mildly improved by using structured interviews and by asking patients to recall and re-state key elements of the discussion. In addition to the ethical imperative of informed consent, it may be that informed patients are less likely to experience medical errors by acting as another layer of protection (as when a patient is able to inform providers about his or her correct medications or the correct surgical procedure he or she is to undergo). More research is needed to establish the best practices to improve informed consent, and to test the impact of such practices on patient safety.

3

Analysing Doctor-Patient Relationship

THE DOCTOR/PATIENT RELATIONSHIP

Purpose: To begin to understand the doctor-patient relationship. In this review, we cover the first five components of the doctor patient relationship listed on page 4.

I. Biopsychosocial Model

A comprehensive approach to patient care in which the biological, psychological, and social aspects of a patient's life are explored. When used, this approach enables the physician to provide more effective treatment. This is in contrast to the biomedical model, where only the biological and medical aspects of a patient's illness are considered relevant information.

II. Empathy

The ability to momentarily experience the feelings of another, i.e. to put oneself in another person's place. This is NOT the same as feeling sorry for a patient, or being supportive.

One must be able to express, transiently, the feelings of another and use those feelings as a tool for understanding that person's subjective experience. Then, one must communicate that understanding to the patient.

It is essential for building a solid therapeutic alliance between the physician and the patient.

Barriers to empathy: Medical students are praised for getting the right answers, not being empathetic. Time is limited. Doctors are often encouraged to use canned, patronizing responses to patient distress, like "Oh, I can see that must be hard for you".

III. Styles of Relating

There are various approaches to the interview:

(1) The quality of the interaction, e.g. warmth vs. detachment

(2) The nature of the communication, e.g. who does the most talking

(3) The decision-making process, e.g. who makes the decisions

There are three physician styles:

(1) Paternalistic or Autocratic Style: Physician makes decisions. Information is provided to patient from physician, physician is dominant in the interview process. Interaction is warm or detached.

(2) Shared Decision-Making Style: Decisions are shared based on expertise of each participant. Information is shared. The physician asks more questions and is less dominant. Interaction is warm.

(3) Consumer-Based Style: Patient makes decisions. Information is provided on the basis of the patient's questions. The patient may dominate the interview. Interaction is warm or detached.

IV. Professional Boundaries

The doctor-patient relationship is fiduciary. The doctor and patient stand in a special relation of trust, confidence, and responsibility in their obligations to each other and to others.

A doctor must keep an appropriate distance from and concern for the patient despite what the patient does. But where does one draw the line about what is the "right" amount of concern?

Most professional organisations state that a sexual relationship between doctor and patient is unethical.

Getting stock tips, giving hugs, holding hands when giving bad news, having sexual relations with former patients, etc...professional organisations are less clear about these and other potential doctor-patient relationship damaging events.

V. Transference, Countertransference

Individuals view one another through distorted lenses that have to do with past experiences and early encounters. Transference: The unconscious displacement of feelings, attitudes, and expectations from important persons in the patient's childhood to current relationships. For example, if a patient has grown up perceiving people around him or her as unhelpful or even harmful, the patient might view his or her physician that way.

Countertransference: The feelings and attitudes of the doctor toward the patient, which could arise from conflicts in the doctor's past. These feelings could also be a response to the patient's projections onto the physician. For example, a young woman might elicit a protective response in a doctor who had helped raise younger female siblings.

Issues of Compliance

— Up to 50 % of patients do not comply
— One study revealed that 1/3 patients complied 1/3 complied somewhat 1/3 were non- compliant
— Can be minimized or exacerbated by the physician and by the quality of the patient-doctor relationship

Factors that Enhance Compliance

1. Good rapport between physician and patient
2. Simple regimens
3. Clear instructions that patient can repeat back to physician
4. Positive feedback for adherence
5. Increased level of distress
6. Decreased waiting room time
7. Increased time with physician
8. Family support and involvement

Identify the reasons why the patient has difficulty adhering to the treatment plan. Examine the factors as they relate to the patient's medical regime, spouse and family, and the doctor-patient relationship. Below are the most common problem patients for physicians. The text goes into detail on each, however, a lot of this was discussed in class and is also outlined in some of the class lecture notes. I tried to give brief summaries on each.

Factors that impede Compliance

1. Low level of subjective distress
2. Denial of illness
3. Poor communication between physician and patient
4. Complex regimens

5. Treatment that is embarrassing of humiliating
6. Outside factors that make compliance difficult
7. Patient's perception that it is beneficial to remain ill
8. Side effects that are significant for the patient

Seductive Patient

— Patient idealizes the doctor taking form in erotic or sexualized transference
— Can be both flattering and disturbing to the physician
— Can evoke [sexual] feelings in the doctor
— Essentially, a doctor cannot stop these feelings. However, it's unethical to act on them and thus, it's not the feelings themselves but what you do with them that may or may not cause trouble

Management

— May need to transfer patient to another doctor
— The doctor can try to sort out their feelings by discussing the situation with colleagues
— It is easier for doctors to deal with these feelings if they have fulfilling lives
— Psychotherapy
— Maintain clear boundaries
— In this case, a psychiatrist was asked to come in. This person assigned a primary doctor and a primary nurse to handle all issues concerning the patient in order to avoid splitting (done by patient).

Example

An attractive woman, experiencing difficulty in her marriage, becomes infatuated with her doctor and expresses a desire to see him outside of the office.

Patient with 1000 Symptoms

— These are somatizing patients

— Appear to be invested in remaining ill

— Doctors get frustrated and angry and often order unnecessary procedures/tests

— These patients show up frequently in general practice; account for 5-10% of patients seen

— The need to be ill is unconscious and patients believe the symptoms are real

Example

Female patient fears she may have a tumor. First, she thinks eye pain = tumor, she is given referral to ophthalmology. Second, she thinks elbow pain = tumor, given referral to orthopedics. Even after seeing a therapist, and making connections between and increase in frequency of symptoms with an increase in stress, she still continues to develop new symptoms and have recurrent fears related to health.

Management

When regular coping mechanisms fail there's a childlike regression- try to understand patient's anger and fear, while helping patient maintain a sense of self control over his environment

Mentally Disturbed Patient

— False assumption that psychotic individuals cannot deal rationally with illness

— Doctors, as well as staff, may feel frightened of these patients

Example

50 y/o man with schizophrenia is diagnosed with colon

cancer. He is admitted to the ward and the staff becomes upset because they are fearful of their safety and feel he should be on the psych floor. They end up avoiding the patient all together. A psychiatrist was called in and found the patient able to understand his illness and able to make decisions regarding his treatment. Therefore, the patient was concerned about why no one was telling him what was going on.

Management

— Provide consistent, competent, non-judgmental care
— Patient does best when seen regularly (once a month) by one personal doctor on long-term basis
— Focus is on management rather than cure
— If able, try to combine psychotherapy

Patient in Hospital Setting

— These patients do well in outpatient setting
— In hospital, they feel robbed of a sense of dignity and personal control
— Patients become childlike
— Will react differently depending on their personality
— Rigid personalities argumentative, non-compliant, denial
— Dependent submissive, helpless
— Paranoid distrustful, depend on 2nd opinions, threaten lawsuits

Example

Self-absorbed man needing a heart valve replace. Suddenly he is threatened by the idea of being weak/sick becomes totally helpless, stays in bed, etc resulting in slow recovery

Management

— A psych consult is appropriate

— As exposure to these patients increases the doctor will become more comfortable and will be able to recognize when a patient is able to discuss the illness and when a patient requires psychiatric care

The Dying Patient

We've pretty much covered this in lecture . . .

— The point of this section is that patient's will deal differently with death.

— Denial may be an effective way for certain patients to continue living.

— The text states that people often die the way they live (but not always). That is, an angry, hostile person will not likely become docile at the end of life.

— There are lots of examples in this section- it seemed intuitive to me you may want to read p.29-33 for more info.

— Patients need to be given control over their situation, be allowed to use their own coping mechanisms, and be treated as part of the living right to the end

— Respect patient's choices regarding living and dying 3 concepts of stress:

(1) stressors - stressful life events

(2) psychological state of stress - feelings of threat, harm, or loss

(3) stress responses - on physiological, psychological, or social levels

- predictors of recovery = psychosocial assests such as strong family ties, flexibility and reliability, realistic goals

- Holmes and Rahe developed the Schedule of Recent Life Events (SRE): The more LCUs (Life Changing Units) were accumulated, the more likely were illnesses of all kinds in a subsequent 2-year period. For example, "death of a spouse" was assigned the highest LCU of 100. Divorce was second highest with an LCU of 73.
- Factors that can either buffer or intensify the stressor

(1) cognitive appraisal of the events - e.g. events that are stressful for one person may not be to another

(2) coping mechanisms (2 types)

  (a) direct action = person tries to alter or master the troubled interaction with the environment (e.g. studying for an exam)

  (b) palliation = reducing affective, visceral, or motor disturbances (e.g. smoking)

(3) social support systems - those with support are protected in crisis from a variety of pathological states

(4) genetic vulnerability - some people have predispositions to stressed-induced physical pathology, some exhibit resilience.

A definition of ethnicity as a concept separate from race, based on three fundamental concepts. These are that:

1. Ethnicity establishes ties between people by providing a reference to common origins
2. Ethnicity implies that members of the collectivity share particular patterns of behaviour and interpersonal interactions.
3. Ethnicity implies that ethnic groups participate with one another in a larger social system

The thesis of this section of the study is that in the context of medical care, it is important for practitioners to become culturally sensitive without reverting to stereotyping. Such sensitivity may facilitate an understanding of how patients present their complaints and respond to treatment approaches.

The authors go on to then present summaries of three theoretical representative ethnic minorities in such broad categories as to (in my opinion) entirely lose sight of their primary thesis. They examine African-American, Hispanic-American, and Asian-American groups.

With respect to African-Americans, they indicate that although African-Americans in general rely on "orthodox biomedicine for their care," that there is a propensity to categorize illnesses as either "natural" or "unnatural". "Unnatural illnesses" are caused by a hex placed upon one by a close relative or friend and cannot be cured by doctors. Hypertension misunderstood as "High-pertension" is used as an example of African-American misunderstanding of standard medical diagnoses and reads (again in my opinion) like bad racist joke. Nonetheless, the salient point of this section of the study is that such patients may perceive changes in diet and weight loss as ineffective recommendations for treatment of hypertension. Without actually citing the Tuskeegee tragedy, the authors acknowledge that African-Americans suspicions of biomedical explanations are in fact rooted in our country's history of racism. This is particularly relevant in the dissemination of public health information to poor black communities.

In their discussion of Hispanic-Americans, the authors acknowledge the tremendous diversity among Spanish-speaking populations in the US, and then focus their discussion on Mexican-Americans and Puerto Rican-

Americans. There are notions of natural and supernatural illnesses and a concept of balance between hot and cold elements. Addressing the issue of language barriers, the authors warn against mislabeling symptoms as "psychotic" when the translation does not appropriately address the notion of anxiety as having a spiritual origin. According to the authors, there are good and evil spirits which may contribute to states of mental health and that these are linked to religious beliefs without conflicting with the predominantly (but not exclusively) Catholic background of most Hispanic-Americans. There are eight philosophical premises cited:

1. Illness can result from strong emotional states
2. Illness can be caused by being out of balance with the environment
3. Patients can be the innocent victims of malevolent forces
4. The body and soul are separable
5. Cure requires participation of the entire family
6. The natural world cannot be distinguished from the supernatural
7. Sickness of a member can bring a family closer
8. A healer should be open and treat you with respect

The Asian-American examples look at the notions of balance again and the life energy of chi. Using the example of Vietnamese culture, the authors explain why a patient who believes that blood is precious would be unhappy about having any drawn - that the relationship between quantity and sustenance are exponential. That is in the order of food blood -> jing chi shen. And it is important to understand that in several languages there is no distinction between the words "food" and "medicine". In order to effectively approach patients, the physician also needs to be aware of his/her own cultural bias. This refers both to the physician's own ethnicity *and* the culture of biomedicine itself. Beware of focussing strictly on treatment rather than alleviating suffering. Biomedical culture in this country may tend to forget that suffering is experienced by persons, not just body. The authors use the example that some cultures (not necessarily our own biomedical one) may value a good death as well as a good life.

The take home:

1. Beliefs influence the interpretation of symptoms and effective communication between the patient and physician.
2. Higher prevalence of disease in minority groups is better understood as social economic situation than a racial one; the stresses of poverty have a significant impact on physical and mental health.
3. The medical community itself has a culture which can be foreign and poorly understood by patients.
4. Don't stereotype, don't draw premature conclusions, use interpreters.

Though some of it seems a long strange tale, this is what it said,

Jared

I. Psychoanalytic Psychology (The first point made is the importance of reading this text as a whole rather than piecemeal, ... whoops.) Based on seeking origins of psychological disturbances.

A. Three aspects of psychoanalytic theory

Methods of investigation, General theories, Methods of Tx

1. One method of investigation: Dreams

a. Dreams represent coded wish fulfillment/ gratification of unconscious infantile wished or urges
b. Uses symbolic thought and irrational thought process (termed "primary process") as occurs throughout the unconscious.
c. Dream work (action of dream activity) x (latent dream content (infantile urges) + day residue (ongoing concerns) + physical sensations during sleep (discomfort or noise)) = manifest dream (remembered dream)
d. Types of dream work (mental activity that makes dreams).

1. Condensation: Large amount of unconscious material in one symbol or image

2. Displacement: Emotionally charged material associated w/ less significant latent content/ lesser events associated w/ more significant latent content

3. Symbolism: unconscious idea represented metaphorically

4. Secondary elaboration: in the dream work, various themes/ images woven into coherent storyline

2. Primary theory of human behaviour

a. Psychic determinism: All psychic events determined by antecedent ones (what about the first one?) and nothing occurs by chance in mental life.
b. Includes topographic model of the mind.

1. Unconscious: contains drives and feelings held out of conscious awareness by countering forces.

2. Preconscious, that part of the unconscious that can be made conscious under directed attention.

3. Conscious: area where "secondary process," occurs, i.e. rational, logical thinking.

4. Various methods of Tx exist for psychiatric disorders.

B. Dynamic or motivational Point of view

1. Using topographical model, behaviour based on instinctual drives of the unconscious

a. Based on the fact that

1. Behaviour not always triggered by external stimuli

2. Behaviour may have causally determined goal-directed (instinctual drive) component

b. Instinctual drives governed by pleasure-unpleasure principle, leading towards activities that provide pleasure, avoiding those that cause pain, with the avoidance of pain being foremost.

c. Instinctual drives require object through which or in regard to which they achieve their aims (e.g. baby at mother's breast)

2. Two primary instinctual drives in psychoanalytic theory

a. Aggressive

b. Sexual/pleasurable

C. Adaptive point of view

1. Humans viewed as a product of an evolution that pre-adapted them to reality.

a. Ego = organ of adaptation

b. Reality and adaptation the "matrix of all behaviour"

D. *Developmental hypotheses*, or genetic point of view (genetic meaning behaviour as a continuum which is genetically dependent on earlier events)

1. Behaviour is a product of two factors:

a. Intrinsic forces: Antecedent to and independent of new experience

b. Experiential factors: Learning and other forms of environmental influence

2. Development a continuum since infancy and occurs in a series of progressions and regressions

3. Fixation: Regression often to a point where patient is fixated, a developmental stage not fully mastered which is retained as a point of emphasis in the personality.

a. Oral stage fixation: Unmet needs for care, nurturing and protection during 0-1 &1/2 yrs. of life lead to general unmeetable hunger for love yet w/ a feeling of being unlovable. Also there are insecure/ mistrustful feelings. *Regression leads to an excessively clinging and dependent state coupled with an unreasonable distrust of the person they have made themselves dependent on.*

b. Anal or sadistic-anal stage: Freud termed this the sadistic-anal stage to emphasize the importance of the aggressive drive at this stage, which occurs at 1&1/2 to 3 yrs. Primary issue is one of control and autonomy, the denying of which leads the child to repress angry feelings. *The fear of expressing emotions leads to an emotional aloofness and constraint termed obsessive compulsive disorder. This disorder is also marked by an attempt to gain love and acceptance by perfection and strict adherence to rules.* Patients regress into indecisiveness, demanding excessive logical explanations at every step in a medical workup as a reason to give up some aspect of the rigid control they exercise on their own decisions, reflecting their unresolved ambivalence over the childhood issue of "should I obey or should I say no." Detailed explanations will avoid powers struggles w/ a regressing anal patient.

c. Phallic or phallic-oedipal stage: Age 3-6, where a boy undergoes the oedipal complex combined w/ castration anxiety leading to the development of the superego. Freud, and I quote, "thought that the girl's first "phallic" impulses were directed towards the mother, and her attention was focused on her clitoris just as the little boys is focused on his penis. Thus the girls first oedipal phase begins with masculine strivings. When the girl discovers the little boys penis, she feels her clitoris inferior and experiences this as a "narcissistic injury," a degrading humiliation that leads both to "penis envy" and blaming of her mother for her plight. ... This leads to relinquishing of the mother as the primary source of love and a turning to the father in hopes that he will provide her with a penis or a baby as a substitute ... her mother now becomes the jealous rival. Whereas, in boys, the oedipal complex is destroyed by the castration complex, in girls, it is made possible and led up to by the castration complex." Because oedipal complex is less repressed in girls due to a lesser threat of genital damage, girls continue to be noticeably more attached to their fathers and more openly in conflict with their mothers. Freud also concluded that the development of the superego was also inadequate in women due to the incomplete resolution of the oedipal complex. This has since been rejected and in the 60s/70s other theories developed which state that the *primary drive of development for girls in this stage is not penis envy but rather based on their primary femininity.*

d. Oedipal defeat: 6-13 yrs Latency Stage. Oedipal complex rejected and identifications of same sex parents solidified.

1. Disturbances in development prior to Oedipal stage lead to distorted oedipal stages.

a. If a girl has cold, unavailable mother, she may turn to intensely towards the father during the oedipal stage. An attention seeking, theatrical, "seductive" little girl routine may develop in adulthood into use of sexuality to gain love and attention to compensate for lack of maternal nurture.

b. If a boy has a cold, rejecting, unavailable father during the oedipal phase who cannot be identified with, boy identifies predominately with the mother leading to the effeminate male or male hysteric. If father subjects the boy to intense teasing, criticism or humiliation, they may develop basic doubts over their own masculinity, adequacy and competence or they may move into a hypermasculine "macho" personality where hyperaggressive, hypersexual, and risk-taking behaviours prove their masculinity.

c. Unresolved Oedipal complexes in both sexes may lead to repeatedly falling in love w/ members of the opposite sex they cannot have or are in some way unavailable or inappropriate. An unresolved oedipal complex may also result in a fear of exceeding same the same sex parent or marring a partner who represents the opposite sex parent and thus "winning" the Oedipal conflict.

BEHAVIOURAL AND SOCIAL LEARNING PSYCHOLOGY

Characteristics of Behavioural Theory

Assumptions:

Terms: the food is called an unconditioned stimulus and the response it elicits is called an unconditioned response or reflex. The bell, a previously neutral stimulus that comes to elicit salivation through conditioning, is called a conditioned stimulus and the response it elicits is a conditioned response. Extinction is when the conditioned stimulus loses the power to elicit the conditioned response by no longer being paired with the unconditioned stimulus. Spontaneous recovery can occur if the two are paired again after a period of time. Generalisation can occur when a stimuli similar to the conditioned stimulus can elicit the conditioned response. Respondent Conditioning and the Development of Emotions John Watson and the "Albert Experiments"—demonstrated that an emotional response and related maladaptive behaviour, such as a phobia, could be acquired through a relatively simple learning process rather than being the result of underlying processes and conflicts that can be neither observed nor studied experimentally.

"Albert Experiments": in this experiment a baby, Albert, was presented with a white rat and initially Albert showed no fear and played affectionately with the rat. Later, upon each presentation with the rat a loud, jarring gong was banged loudly which greatly frightened Albert. Albert began to associate the gong with the rat and Albert cried whenever he was shown the rat. He began to generalize his fears to anything white and furry and cried when presented with anything vaguely resembling the rat: white teddy bear, white fur coat, etc.

Conditioned emotional responses can be positive or negative:

— Negative: Albert's fear of white furry objects

— Positive: the sound of a lover's voice

Operant Conditioning/ Internal Conditioning

A. B.F. Skinner

— in operant conditioning, an animal or person "operates" on the environment and produces a change, a consequence for the behaviour.

— Ex: bird pushes a lever and receives food.

Consequences are defined in terms of their effect on behaviour. If the effect is to strengthen or increase behaviour, the event is reinforcing. If the behaviour is decreased or weakened by the event, it is punishing.

B. Reinforcement: the procedure of increasing the probability of a behaviour occurring by the contingent delivery of a reinforcing event that follows the behaviour.

— reinforcers may be positive or negative depending on whether the consequence entails the presentation or removal of some event.

Example: One patient may take medication as ordered because doing so is associated with either improved physical status or attention and praise from family members and the physician-Positive reinforcement. Another patient may comply with the physician's order because taking the medication results in the termination or avoidance of unpleasant physical symptoms.

Schedules of Reinforcement

If a response has been reinforced continuously, then it will extinguish more rapidly than if it has been reinforced on an intermittent basis. Behaviour maintained by intermittent schedules is said to be more resistant to extinction.

Example: The continuous complaining of the patient described above will decrease more rapidly if sympathy is consistently withheld vs. intermittently withheld.

Punishment

Positive punishment-the contingent presentation of an event immediately after the occurrence of behaviour with a resulting decrease in the probability of that behaviour.

Negative punishment-contingent *removal of a positive reinforcer* with a resultant reduction in the future occurrence of the response. But increase in probability of behaviour.eg. time out for kids.

Example: Positive punishment-criticism from one's boss for tardiness to one's job. Negative punishment-losing part of one's wages for the time missed from work (or losing one's job). Time out from positive reinforcement is frequently used as a negative punisher for child misbehaviour.

Ex: child is sent to "the corner" following a misbehaviour (time out from positive reinforcers-toys, T.V., play).

Developing New Behaviour

A. Shaping: the starting point is to identify behaviour that is already occurring that resembles the desired behaviour and to reinforce it. The procedure of differentially reinforcing closer and closer approximations to the final target behaviour is called the *method of successive approximations.*

B. Imitation: We acquire a great deal of behaviour by simply observing others and imitating their behaviours. Modeling is a very powerful means of learning new behaviour.

C. Extinction: In extinction, the reinforcer that has maintained a response no longer follows the behaviour and the behaviour decreases and is eliminated.

Example: Chronic pain patients may complain excessively about physical discomfort for which there is no medical cure. Such complaints are frequently maintained by the attention and sympathy when complaining occurs. The behaviour to be eliminated depends on the schedule of reinforcement.

Social Learning or Social Cognitive Theory

This theory is based on the interaction of mental, behavioural and personal factors in the learning process. An important factor in the learning process is modeling.

Modeling: learning that occurs by observing others and the consequences of other behaviours.

Antecedents

— Consequences are important in explaining operant behaviour; antecedents of behaviour are also important in explaining behaviour.

— People behave a certain way in presence of certain stimuli/situations.

— This is due to discrimination training: in presence of certain stimuli, behaviour is *reinforced*; in presence of different stimuli, behaviour is *extinguished*.

— Example = Two parents can react differently to a child's tantrums...child will only perform tantrums in presence of parent that responds to this behaviour...that parent can actually serve to cause this behaviour (since he/she is a reinforcer).

— *Reinforcement* of behaviour is done by the discriminative stimulus (SD).

Non-reinforcement of behaviour is done by S-delta (S).

— Discriminated behaviour: when behaviour is more

likely to occur w/ SD than in its absence (stimulus control is thus established).

— Person may not be aware of discriminated behaviour/ stimulus control

— Example = When a patient complains more about his/her condition in the presence of another person than when alone.

— To facilitate development of discriminative behaviour, 2 stimuli may be presented together...one is faded over time.

— Example = Modeling of a behaviour is done along with directions for that given behaviour; eventually, the modeling is faded out and directions are used to perform behaviour.

— Generalisation: now, want behaviour to occur in presence of new/different stimuli.

— This is done by generalisation training: reinforcement of behaviour in presence of other stimuli until all members of that stimuli class are associated with the given behaviour.

— Example = practicing being assertive with one friend until you can be assertive with your entire group of friends.

Problems with the use of Negative Reinforcement

1. Punishing agent often models aggressive behaviour, verbally or physically, and teaches the youngster that aggression is an acceptable means of dealing with people.

2. Punishment generates emotional behaviour and more intense verbal or physical activity. Ex: temper tantrums, etc.

3. People learn to avoid punishment instead of the moral basis behind the consequence.

4. Negative emotional responses are conditioned when aversive controls are used. For example, a youngster learns to dislike homework because nagging and criticism are used to keep the child on task.

5. Punishment produces response suppression, which can generalize to other behaviours.

Principle of Reciprocal Inhibition

— Different behaviours can be reciprocal inhibiting: occurrence of one behaviour inhibits the other.

— Example = Cat was shocked in cage when given food...cat developed anxiety to cage and did not feed, despite extreme hunger...neurotic behaviour generalized to situations similar to initial experiment...*Wolpe hypothesized that since feeding was inhibited by anxiety, that anxiety may be inhibited by feeding*...feeding was induced in cage...eventually anxiety disappeared...conclusion: cat cannot be both anxious and engaged in feeding.

— Behaviour therapy developed from related work.

— *Systematic desensitisation: pairing deep muscle relaxation w/imagined scenes in a graded fashion from least —> most provoking.*

— *Response to anxiety-provoking stimulus is reconditioned w/relaxation...anxiety is inhibited.*

— *Such reconditioning is based on principle of reciprocal inhibition and substantiated by experiments.*

Social Learning/Social Cognitive Theory

— Self-regulation (Bandura's social cognitive theory)

— Self-direction = important aspect of theory

— 3 processes of self-regulation:

(1) Self-observation/monitoring: "In order to obtain info. to establish standards of behaviour and to judge current behaviour relative to those standards, one must observe relative dimensions of one's behaviour with some regularity and accuracy."

Dysfunction = Depressed people *negatively distort* their perceptions/recollections.

(2) Self-evaluation/judgment: "This process entails evaluation of behaviour in relation to internalized personal standards and other points of reference such as peers or a normative group as well as consideration of the value of the performance."

Dysfunction = Depressed mood due to negative appraisal of performance, with failure attributed to lack of ability rather than situational factors; accomplishments devalued in relation to others.

(3) Self-reaction/directs and motivates behaviour: "Individuals can evaluate their behaviour positively or negatively and reward or punish the performance."

Dysfunction = Depressed people more likely to punish.

— Self-efficacy (Bandura)

"Perceived self-efficacy is defined as people's judgments of their capabilities to organise and execute courses of action required to attain designated types of performances. It is concerned not with the skills one has but with the judgments of what one can do with whatever skills one possesses."

— The greater one's self-efficacy, the more likely one will persist in face of difficulty.

— 4 source of info. for self-efficacy:

(1) Success experiences vs. failures.

(2) Vicarious experiences in which others are seen to be capable.

(3) Verbal persuasion (psyching oneself up)

(4) Physiological state indicates susceptibility to failure.

— Useful for examining anxiety disorders.

— Expectations regarding outcome/efficacy cause fear/ avoidance...rather than fear causing avoidance.

Clinical Applications: Cognitive and Behavioural Therapies

— Application of lab-based psych. principles for changing behaviour (operant and/or respondent conditioning).

— Cognitive-behavioural therapy: treatment with both behavioural (i.e. social skills training) and cognitive (i.e. expectancies) components.

— Cognitive Behaviour Modification (Meichenbaum)

— Same principles that govern observable behaviour also can be applied to modify private events/cognitions ("self-talk")...thereby altering behaviour/emotions.

2. Procedures:

(1) Self-instructional training = individuals learn what they say to themselves in problem situations and correct it.

(2) Stress inoculation training = acquisition of coping skills.

— Rational-emotive Therapy (RET) (Ellis)

— Focuses on changing patterns of thinking directly;

based on assumption that one's interpretations of events produce emotional consequences.

— Cognitive Therapy (Beck)

— Person's perception of events causes emotional distress.

— Negative self-schema developed in childhood...carries into adulthood.

Therapy Techniques

(1) Contingency management: application of reinforcement/punishment to change behaviour.

(2) Parent training: instruction in contingency management skills.

(3) Contingency Contract: contingencies mutually agreed upon and written down.

(4) Social skills training: systematic instruction/training in a communication area using behavioural principles.

(5) Exposure to fear-provoking stimuli: treatment for many anxiety disorders.

(6) Systematic desensitisation: gradual imaginal exposure.

(7) Imaginal flooding: indirect exposure in a prolonged/ abrupt fashion; patient imagines scenario until anxiety decreases (used for post-traumatice stress disorders).

(8) Response prevention: not allowing patient to engage in behaviours that serve an anxiety-reductive function...forces patient to confront anxiety.

(9) Relaxation techniques: progressive muscle relaxation, diaphragmatic breathing, visualisation techniques.

(10) Biofeedback: promotes self-regulation of physiological responses.

(11) Cognitive Restructuring: alterations in patterns of thinking.

(12) Problem-solving skills training: good for impulsive behaviours.

(13) Stress-management training

Behavioural Medicine

— Application of behaviour principles/technology to medical/health-related problems.

Prevention of Illness and Disease

— Primary Prevention = intervention to prevent onset of illness/injury.

— Secondary Prevention = promoting healthy behaviours after an illness has been diagnosed.

— Helping patients cope with invasive procedures/ painful treatments.

Contributions of Behavioural Approach

(1) Entails formulation of specific, individualized goals for treatment, consisting of objectively defined/ observable behaviours.

(2) Self-evaluative; empirical demonstration of effectiveness/identification of limits of interventions are a committment of the field.

(3) Interventions implemented/assessed in patient's natural environment; less time-consuming/expensive.

Comparisons of the Behavioural and Psycholanytic Models

— Multiple differences b/w the two models.

— At least one similarity: Determinism... psychoanalysts/behaviourists both posit causes for behaviour that do not include free will.

— Psychoanalytic theory in a nutshell:

— Behaviour symbolic of underlying/intrapsychic processes; neurotic behaviour = symptom of unconscious conflict.

— Treatment: focus on understanding underlying processes, rather than on behaviour/symptoms.

— Early experiences very significant.

— Subjective; therapist uses inference/interpretation; based on case histories.

— Mechanisms of change unobservable.

— Behavioural theory in a nutshell:

— Behaviour is focus of treatment.

— Behaviour is determined by reinforcement history, current contingencies, genetic endowment (not by intrapsychic processes).

— Observable environmental events analysed.

— Contemporary (not historical) factors emphasized in explaining/changing behaviour (by operant and/ or classical conditioning).

— Objective; based on empirical method.

The Mid-life Transition

— between ages 35 & 55 most adults realise they've reached the midpt. of their lifespan

— they realise they no longer have most of their life ahead of them

— they see life as a "whole" w/it's boundaries and limits

— confrontation of these limits can be the basis of a thorough readjustment of self

— before the midpt. of life, most adults are in "consolidation"

— a period in which they continue makng progress toward personal and professional goals w/little time for introspection

— a mild crisis/ trauma can interrupts this illusory state

— new realities appear: signs of physical aging, onset of menopause, diminished sexual desire, "sandwiching due to simultaneous responsibility for kids and aging parents, plateauing of advancement & work

— 1st major medical illness (i.e. myocardial infarction) or death of a peer in their prime causes the individual to confront their own mortality

— disillusionment of youthful fantasies is necessary to make the transition to mature adulthood

— individuals undergo life review; reassess the past & present and set new limits

— ultimate goal: new integration of self , in which a # of conflicting polarities (love-hate, success-failure, etc.) are reconciled

— Mid-life crisis: block or maladaptive response to mid-life transition

Bereavement

— loss plays a role in every life transition

— Bereavement: specific reaction to loss of a person to whom one has been attached. This is largely a self-limited psychological process that unfolds through a series of stages from initiation to resolution

— to overcome any major loss (ex. of spouse, child, parent, body part) one must review & relive the lost relationship

— Initial reaction - some form of denial
— some people show absence of emotion, this is due to shock/psychic numbness
— consequence: grief experience is post-poned or never reached
— signs of grieving:
— intense emotion, including mixtures of sadness, tearfulness, maybe rage
— preoccupied w/their own feeling & inner experience
— quasihallucinatory phenomena (ex. hearing voice or seeing the departed)
— important task in grief - coming to terms w/ ambivalent feeling
— bereavement exaggerates normal ambivalenc & might stop the individual from working through negative feeling (b/c it's wrong "to speak ill of the dead")
— some degree of guilt is the normal aftermath of grief
— some bereaved split their ambivalence by overidealizing lost person or blaming their loss on a scapegoat
— many malpractice law suits originate when physicians used as scapegoats
— this prevents/prolongs resolution of grief & mourning
— Detachment
— facilitated by reality testing which occurs everytime you think dead person is alive & must remember that they no longer are
— people's who's grieving is incomplete believe the dead live in another world or as ghosts, or are

looking over them (guardian angels)

- Public mourning (funerals, wakes, etc.)
- helps bereaved remember the dead & begin to relinquish their attachments
- to some extent, this has been transferred from religious to medical setting
- physicians can use their position & skills to guide bereaved through stages of grief; they lend support to the legitimicy of grief and counteract bereaved individual's fear that something is wrong w/them
- Pathological bereavement - one or more features of grieving process become exaggerated and/or fixated
- Ex. absent grief, chronic bereavement, excessive guilt, loss of reality
- w/o treatment, these conditions tend to "take on a life of their own"
- Psychotherapy can serve as a catalyst to the grieving process & help unearth blocks in the search for a healthier degree of resolution

The Transition to Late Life

- major task old age - enhance & maintain sense of inner emotional integrity in face of increasing external threats to health, financial status, external support systems
- external supports that aid in sense of identity: attractive & healthy body, social network & family, some authority in the work place
- threats to emotional integrity may be conquered by getting new external supports, experiments with new methods of self-validation & psychotherapy
- relinquishing power & authority stimulate search

for new sources of productivity & creativity. This transition is usually marked by retirement

- what the elderly may lose, they regain in symbolic forms (ex. figurehead)
- older age transition requires construction of new social networks to replace previous ones

Battle for Integrity

- most common threat to sense of integrity of older person is isolation
- elderly especially vulnerable to stimulus deprivation resulting from decreased sensory acuity (vision, hearing, taste, smell)
- as these inner resources decline, importance of external supports increase
- sometimes older people view sickness and death as a test of their personal integrity & inner resource

The Battle for Integrity

- Physicians need to sensitize themselves to patients' needs to:
- Participate in the process of recovery
- Use their own adaptive measures to maintain a sense of autonomy and control
- A physician may not oppose eccentric and unorthodox approaches to self-tx by patient if they cause no harm and add to patient's feeling of being more in control

Death and Dying

- The approach of death may lead to
- feelings of inner continuity
- greater intensity to present moment and greater

depth of self-awareness (because future is foreclosed)

- feel nearer to beginning, or to the cycle of generations (being at the end of the lifecycle)
- Having come full circle, patient may approach end of life with sense of mystery, interest in the transcendent (expressed through increased involvement with religion and larger social issues)
- However, the encounter with one's own impending death (especially before the expected end of lifespan) is an emotionally traumatic event that often exceeds bereavement.
- The disturbing quality of impending death is due to 3 factors:

  (1) We want control of our destiny. Death is a threat to that in our minds. We find it difficult to grasp the idea of our own nonexistence.

  (2) Like the monsters of our childhood, primitive fears of death may transform death into a horrifying specter. Death evokes a series of infantile emotional danger situations, including, loss of the object's love, castration, other forms of physical mutilation, abandonment by parental caretakers (often symbolized as God).

  (3) Western culture of past 100 years has produced a massive denial of death. Study of Hiroshima survivors showed how excessive exposre to death can undermine and destroy much of the meaningfulness of life. A certain degree of adaptive denial ("nothing bad can happen to me") can actually improve life expectance in male patients with myocardial infarction. Societal denial, however, placed death outside the realm of the normal lifecycle, excluding it from everyday

awareness...thus when death appears it if often an alien unwelcome intruder.

— Death was not always viewed as an "extraordinary" event. During the Middle Ages, people met death with a sense of resignation and acceptance, probably due to the universality of religion and frequent exposure to death. Also, death was expected.

— Revival of interest in death and dying in medical settings (partly catalyzed by Elizabeth Kubler-Ross in the 60's) led to rediscovery of the latter attitude. Kubler-Ross wrote that the encounter with death was a developmental process not unlike other life transitions. In the Leo Tolstoy novel The Death of Ivan Ilych, the encounter with death had most of the elements of a midlife crisis. The encounter involved a lengthy and painful task of self-reassessment and realignment. Also, Kubler Ross described the acceptance of death-related tasks as denial and isolation, anger, bargaining, depression, and acceptance——which are somewhat analogous to the stages of bereavement, in this case, loss of one's self.

— The first death of a patient is a painful experience for med students as it puts to the test one's attitudes toward death. The first death may reveal that they were motivated to become a doctor by altruistic "rescue fantasies". Some physicians align with society's recent prevailing attitude of denial, which is "life at any cost". Most ideally will expand their definition of medical success to include helping dying patients and their families come to terms with and to achieve a dignified, painless, and peaceful death.

— A doctor's attitude toward death can be revealed in the approach taken in informing a patient of a terminal prognosis. A goal of the physician is to respect and enhance the patient's freedom to define this task in his or her own way. The physician must avoid any preestablished or prescribed policy in this regard. Physicians who never inform their patients of their specific medical situation, or who inform the terminal patients with all of the details, may interfere with freedom of choice for some patients.

— Some patients may not want to know the specific prognosis of their illness. Some may not want to know their diagnosis, or may prefer to discuss it in vague terms. While this attitude shows some denial, it indicates a certain choice of how to approach death. These patients approach death as an invisible horizon, always just beyond their range of vision. They focus on tasks of improving their situation and wish for improvement or for a miracle cure...which allows them to maintain their denial, live with hope, bolster optimism. The point is that the doctor is not in a position to know beforehand what path will be chosen by an individual patient.

— Extreme denial may place a burden on the patient's family and business by resulting in lack of preparation of a will and of other planning for the future. A will commits individuals to the serious consideration of their own death and its consequences for others.

— For many death in the abstract is not the main source of anxiety. Patients may want reassurance, not that the physician will save them, but that he or she will stay with them as an ally, partner, and consultant right to the end. Often, the dying patient's most haunting fear is of being left alone. Patients want reassurance from the physician that he or she will not allow the patient to be overwhelmed by pain and physical suffering.

— A case study of a 50 year old man with terminal metastatic colon cancer revealed the following:

— The patient was observed with behaviour and concerns that were due to partial psychological regression. Most of the time, he acted like a mature man trying to work through his feelings about his impending death....hence tearfulness due to the mourning process. However, he had been asking his wife to bring him huge quantities of his favourite, nutritious foods. In order to deal with the inescapable ending of his life, he had shrunk his temporal horizon to encompass only his next meal. Also, he saw his wife and the staff nurses as all-powerful "mother" figures who held the power of life and death over him. He felt as though they could keep him alive or they could kill him with poison introduced into his IV line. The psychiatrist assigned had to support and encourage the staff to accept the patient's unique approach to death. The psychiatrist listened to the patient and tolerated his partial behavioural regressions without criticism.

— In the course of the developmental process, many patients come to conceive of their encounter with death in terms of a metaphor, i.e., a fight that's been lost, a journey culminated closure of life, a return to the beginning of the lifecycle, a profound rest. Many patients may think of death as a transition. For example, one patient dreamed about his death as a move from his old house to a new one.

— One aspect of the developmental process of death that sets it apart from other developmental processes is the need for a more thoroughgoing divestment from all of life's attachments.

— The most fundamental fear of patients is not necessarily death itself, but the fear of being alone, abandoned, in pain, and helpless in the process of dying. The physician may play a powerful supportive role for the patient in a terminal illness by:

— Reassure patients that they won't be abandoned. Physicians who withdraw maybe can't emotionally tolerate the idea of death, or react to the patient's terminal illness as a failure to "save". This feeling on the part of the physician may be derived from the physician's fear of death, discomfort with dealing with the emotional pain of bereavement, or a sense of helplessness and failure.

— The second major fear of patients is the fear of feeling helpless in the process of dying. Physicians may provide comforting reassurance that everything will be done to assist patients in their care to ensure as much autonomy as possible.

— Finally, physicians may provide reassurance that the patient will not be allowed to be in significant pain.

Choice in Adult Development: The Transitions as Crossroads

Scenarios: Each individual confronted with a fateful choice

— continue as artist or pursue a more business-oriented career

— continue career as primary caregiver or switch to a

consulting practice - Decisions in the lifecycle about relationships are as important as those involving job and career

— two men both considering separating from their wives

— a schizoid man finally took the plunge and successfully asked and took a woman on a date. His decision was a conscious effort to break out of his self-imposed prison on isolation.

— Ultimately, it's not just a question of "this job or that job," or this relationship or that relationship, but of this or that life path. The individual must choose among various "lifelines." Committing oneself to one choice often means changing the direction of an entire life, and in some cases, altering one's destiny and sense of identity. Adult transitions involve more than just a change from one stage to another. They can be crossroads in the lifecycle, an opportunity for choice against the background of inevitable biological and psychosocial change.

— Most midlife and later choices do not necessarily involve dramatic changes in behaviour. Radical changes in lifestyle in the midlife transition are more the exception than the rule. Some changes may be more symbolic and on a smaller scale (i.e. smoking habit vs. career shift). Some important choices may involve no changes in outward behaviour. The act of choosing does not require change for the sake of change.

— "Refocusing on life choices" is part of the lifecycle stage, which also includes accepting the absolute inevitability of death, yet even in the face of death, a wide range of human choice is not lacking, including the option of rejecting or accepting the finality of death.

— In later life, some individuals feel robbed of the idealized life they fantasize they would have had "if only they had made different choices." The midlife and late-life transition offers many people real or symbolic second chances, however, some adults are blocked from doing so by an idelogy that 'failure is my fate," which they have developed to justify their condition. They may consciously and unconsciously minimize the influence of their choices in shaping their lives.

— Psychotherapy for adults, including the elderly, may be looked upon as a kind of laboratory for the making of choices (help reconsider past situations as the result of choices unwittingly made or evaded, get new perspective). Psychotherapy can help during their development and aid in their efforts to negotiate more successful adult transitions.

Biomedical Model: Suggests that treating one's specific physical pathology is synonymous with treating the patient, which ignores the fundamental truth that all illness simultaneously affects the mind and the body. For example, it defines peptic ulcer disease as the anatomical end product of gastric hypersecretion, implying that definitive treatment consists solely of appropriate medication and dietary restrictions, failing to address specific psychosocial issues affecting and affected by the patient's ulcer.

Biopsychosocial Model (Engel): Theoretical construct that assesses a person within the distinctive context of supports and stressors affecting his/her daily functioning. Requires an understanding of interplay among each patient's medical disorder, intrapsychic life, and the positive and negative impact of his/her external environment. Can determine the course of the following:

1. genesis and exacerbation of an illness
2. mind-body interactions in specific physiological, endocrinological, and immunological processes, as well as generalized stress reactions.
3. one's willingness and ability to cooperate in prescribed care
4. physical illness can precipitate a variety of abnormal psychological states that adversely influence the disease process, or reach a degree of severity so intense that they become more threatening to patients than their original medical disorder.

Illness Dynamics: The relationship among one's biological status (e.g., genetic constitution and physical pathology), emotional makeup, and the supports and stresses of a social matrix (confluence of biologic, psychologic, and social aspects). Represents the patient's understanding of a specific disease during a particular period of life. Illness dynamics incline one to assess all illness-related information in light of singular values, wishes, needs, and fears, ultimately causing the patient to perceive, assess, and defend against the loss of health in a highly subjective manner. This may significantly affect the patient's ability to cope with the disease.

Cultural Attitudes

Grief Process and Illness: Grief reaction is occurs when patients mourn the loss of their previous healthier functioning. The working through of these emotions is analogous to grieving for a loved one. Grieving entails recognition of the good and bad associated with a particular loss, which prompts a series of feeling states - *denial, anxiety, anger, and depression* - that a person must progress through before resolving those emotions and coming to terms with a temporary or permanent health impairment.

The emotional response to a myocardial infarction illustrates this process:

Denial - Patients often attempt to deny reality of precordial pain by minimizing the symptom or explaining it away as indigestion, myalgia, or bronchitis.

Anxiety - When denial recedes as persisting angina underscores medical reality and precipitates a host of intense feelings. There is immediate anxiety about prospect of dying, discomfort of acute treatment, and need to abdicate considerable responsibility and autonomy to anonymous caretakers.

Anger - Once patients feel secure they will survive, they direct their resentments of being sick globally and toward specific targets

Depression - Anger abates, and patient develops a growing a depression, characterized by emotional, behavioural, and cognitive changes that reflect their extreme preoccupation with real and potential losses brought on by the heart attack.

One's illness dynamics facilitate or impede the grief process.

Abnormal Illness Responses: *Patient becomes mired in one stage of the grief process, promoting a preoccupation with feelings characteristics of that phase, thereby preventing resolution of the varied emotions precipitated by loss of heath; analogous to pathological grief.*

The most common abnormal responses include the following:

Denial Response - Persistent denial is often reflected in noncompliance with therapeutic regimen, which my commence immediately after a medical crisis (e.g., refusal to maintain bedrest while recuperating from an MI) and continue throughout a chronic illness (e.g., continued smoking in a patient with chronic obstructive pulmonary disease).

Anxiety Response - Patient becomes hypersensitive about illness; such absorption with one's physical status greatly detracts from all other aspects of life, progressively displacing former pleasures with a debilitating angst.

Anger Response - Engages in overt and covert struggles with people in their lives, which fosters a progressive isolation from necessary support and undermines their medical care.

Depression Response - Causes such withdrawal that the patient is unwilling or unable to provide an adequate medical history or report objective and subjective responses to a therapeutic regimen. Interferes with normative healing processes by debilitating neurovegetative symptoms (e.g., anorexia), a diminished immunological response, passive abandonment of a will to live, or even purposeful self-destructive behaviours.

Dependency Response - Patient becomes excessively dependent on healthcare personnel or relatives and may haphazardly adhere to prescribed therapies to that caretaker must then compensate for patient's self-neglect by providing an even greater degree of care.

The Doctor-Patient Relationship in the Psychological Care of the Medically Ill

Psychotherapy - can be broadly classified as the following:

1. *Supportive* (anxiety-suppressing) - preserve the patient's psychological status quo. Required with

medically ill patients if they manifest symptoms of a pathological illness response. Administered by psychiatrist or other mental health professional.

2. *Introspective* (anxiety-provoking) - heighten insight by obliging the patient to explore painful memories and emotional experiences. Effected by primary caretakers, designed to help patients identify and ventilate intense feelings precipitated by ill health.

The biopsychosocial approach, which acknowledges the inextricable link between mind and body, requires an understanding of patients' illness dynamics and the application of standard psychotherapeutic principles to medical management. A necessary requirment for this treatment approach is *empathic* communication between patients and their caretakers. This process involves transiently identifying with the patient; that is, imagining what it would be like to be in his or her situation, then "pulling back" as an understanding, more objective yet empathic observer.

Hollis (1964) describes four categories of *intervention*:

1. sustaining procedures (e.g., demonstration of a desire to help)
2. procedures of direct influence (e.g., offering suggestions and advice)
3. facilitation of catharsis (e.g., sanctioning the expression of emotions)
4. guidance concerning the day-to-day implications of illness (e.g., urging the return to work or a change in one's living situation)

In establishing dynamic partnership between doctor and patient, need *informed consent*, which rests on four basic elements:

1. provision of information to patients concerning recommended actions, benefits, risks, and alternatives of medical treatments
2. assurance that patients understand the information provided concerning various medical treatments
3. assurance that the patients' decisions concerning medical treatment are made voluntarily, in the absence of coercion
4. eliciting patients' consent via active authorisation, as opposed to passive assent.

DOCTORS, WHAT TO CONSIDER WHEN CHOOSING AHA RECOMMENDATION

We don't provide referral to physicians, cardiac surgeons, nurses, physician's assistants, nutritionists, physical therapists or occupational therapists. However, we offer these suggestions to help you consider options.

Where Can I find names of Qualified Doctors?

— Ask your family, friends, other doctors or your local medical society for recommendations. Then find out more about those recommended.

— Ask the doctors' offices whether they're covered by your medical insurance plan. You can also ask for a list of approved doctors from your insurance company or your employer's health plan administrator.

— Check the doctors' credentials in the American Medical Directory, the Directory of American Specialists, or other professional directory at your local library. Board-certified doctors have completed specific training in their fields and passed required tests.

— Find out where the doctors' offices are located and

with what hospitals they're affiliated.

- If you need to be treated for a specific condition, find out how much experience each recommended doctor has with it. Ask the doctor or the doctor's office how many people he or she has treated with your condition.

What should I consider after meeting with a doctor?

- How confident and comfortable did you feel with the doctor?
- Did the doctor listen to your concerns and answer your questions in a way you can understand?
- Did the doctor explain your medical situation and describe your treatment options in a way you can understand?

Your relationship with a doctor is long term. Be aware that good communication is a two-way process. It may take several visits to develop a good rapport.

QUESTIONS TO ASK YOUR DOCTOR

Many people may have questions for their doctors about tests, surgery and other procedures, therapy and recovery, drug treatment, risk factors and lifestyle changes. Here are examples of common questions; the topics are in alphabetical order.

About Diet after Heart Attack, Stroke or Surgery

- What foods should I eat?
- What foods should I limit?
- How do I read food labels?
- What are some cooking tips for me?
- What about eating out?
- What can I eat at fast-food restaurants?

— How can I control the portions?
— How much salt may I eat?

About Blood Cholesterol

— What do my cholesterol numbers mean?
— What is my goal cholesterol level?
— How often should I have my levels checked?
— How does exercise affect my cholesterol levels?
— What type of foods should I eat?
— Will I need cholesterol-lowering medicine?
— How long will it take to reach my cholesterol goals?

About High Blood Pressure

— What should my blood pressure be?
— What are my options in controlling high blood pressure?
— How often should my blood pressure be checked?
— What about home blood pressure monitors?
— Should I use blood pressure machines at stores?
— How does exercise affect my blood pressure?
— What's my daily sodium (or salt) limit?
— Is there sodium in the medicine I take?
— Will I need to take blood pressure medicine?
— Will I always have to take medicine?
— Why do I need to lose weight?

About Drug Treatment

— Will I need to take medicine?
— What kind of medicine should I take?
— Will my insurance cover this medication?

— Can I take the generic form of the medicine?
— What should I know about the medicine?
— What are the side effects?
— How do I know if it's working?
— How can I remember when to take medicine?
— What if I forget to take a medicine?
— Should I avoid any foods or other medicines?
— Can I drink alcohol?
— How long will I need to take my medicine?
— Will I have to keep taking medicine?

About the Hospital (Before Surgery or Procedure)

— When do I check in?
— What will happen before the (surgery, procedure)?
— How long will it take?
— Where can my family wait for me?
— What effects (temporary or permanent) will the surgery have on me?
— What is the doctor's experience in performing this procedure?
— What medicines will be prescribed (short term/long term)?
— For how long will I have to rest at home after surgery?

About a Pacemaker or Implanted Defibrillator

— Does the shock hurt?
— How long will my batteries last?
— How do I know if it's working?
— When can I take showers and baths?

— Can I swim?
— What equipment or devices should I avoid?
— Can my arrhythmia be cured?

About Physical Activity After Stroke, Heart Attack or Surgery

— Why is physical activity important?
— Can I exercise? When?
— Can I play sports?
— What are the best types of activities for me?
— How much activity do I need?
— Can I have sex?

About Physical Therapy and Rehabilitation

— When do I start rehabilitation?
— How often should I go to rehab?
— Is it covered by my health insurance?
— How long will I need therapy?
— What happens when my rehab programme stops?

About Quitting Cigarettes and Tobacco

— What can I do to stop the cravings?
— How many minutes do cravings last?
— What about a nicotine patch or gum?
— After I quit, when will the urges stop?
— What if I start gaining weight?
— How can I keep from gaining weight?
— How can family and friends help?
— What if I slip and go back to tobacco?
— How long will it take to reduce my risk?

— What do I do if a nicotine patch or gum doesn't work?

About Recovery at Home (After Heart Attack, Stroke or Surgery)

— Can leaving the hospital cause mixed feelings?

— Will I need special transportation or equipment?

— Should I stay in bed?

— How much activity can I do?

— How can my family help me?

— Can I get financial assistance?

— Can I get emotional assistance?

— Can I get in-home assistance for daily tasks?

— What type of diet should I eat?

— What about medicine?

— Will my (aphasia, chest pains, weakness, etc.) go away?

— When should I call my doctor?

— Are my feelings normal?

— What if I stay depressed?

— Can I have sex?

— How soon can I drive?

— When can I go back to work?

— When should I schedule a visit to the doctor?

— How can I prevent another attack?

— What changes should I make in my lifestyle?

About Surgery or Procedures

— Will I need surgery?

— Why do I need it?

— What is the surgery or procedure like?
— How is it done?
— What are the risks?
— Could I have a stroke or heart attack during surgery?
— What are the alternatives?
— Will I need this procedure or surgery again?
— What should my family know?

About Symptoms and Warning Signs

— How can I tell a heart attack from angina?
— How is a heart attack different from a stroke?
— How is a TIA different from a stroke?
— What should I do if I have any of the symptoms of a stroke or heart attack?
— Where can I or someone in my family take a CPR class?

About Recovery in the Hospital (After Stroke, Heart attack or Surgery)

— What happens after surgery?
— How soon can my family visit?
— Will there be pain or fever?
— What are the ICU and CCU?
— What happens in the ICU and CCU?
— What are the tubes and wires for?
— Can I see the monitors?
— What does it mean if an alarm goes off?
— What feelings can arise in the ICU?
— When will I leave the ICU?
— How long will the breathing tube stay in?

— What happens when I leave the ICU?
— What can be done to help in recovery?
— How soon can I get out of bed?
— What is a good sleeping position?
— When can I eat and drink?
— What about bathing?
— When will my (chest, head, neck, leg, etc.) heal?
— What about medicine?
— How long will the pain last?
— When do I start rehabilitation?
— How long do I stay in the hospital?
— What should my family know?

About Weight Control

— Why are weight control and physical activity important?
— How often should I check my weight?
— How much weight should I lose?
— How fast should I lose weight?
— What diet guidelines should I follow?
— What are the best types of physical activities for me?
— How much physical activity do I need to do?
— How much weight gain is too much?
— How can family and friends help?
— How do I find a dietitian to help me develop a good, long-term weight-loss plan?

About Tests for Heart or Brain Function

— Why do I need it?

— How is it done?
— Will it hurt?
— What will the test show?
— How soon will I get the results?
— What is monitored during the test?
— What equipment is used?
— Is there a risk?
— Could it give me a heart attack or stroke?
— What are the alternatives?
— Will my artificial heart valve cause problems?
— Could my implanted pacemaker cause problems?
— Will I need more tests?

SECOND MEDICAL OPINIONS

AHA Recommendation

We don't make referrals to physicians, cardiac surgeons, nurses, physician's assistants, nutritionists, physical therapists or occupational therapists. We can offer these suggestions to help people seeking second (or third or more) opinions:

When should I get another medical opinion?

— If your insurance company requires it before it will cover your treatment
— If there are several options for treating your condition, or you want to know if there are other options
— If the treatment your doctor recommends has significant risk
— If the treatment will greatly affect your lifestyle, work or family

— If you feel rushed to make a decision and want more information

— If you don't have full confidence in the recommended treatment or in the doctor

Doctors expect (and many managed care plans require) their patients to seek other opinions. Don't worry about hurting the doctor's feelings when you ask for one.

How Can I Get Another Medical Opinion?

— Your doctors may refer you to other doctors or specialists.

— Ask friends or relatives who've been treated for the same condition.

— Ask for a list of approved doctors from your medical insurance company or your employer's health plan administrator.

— Call your local medical society.

— Check the American Medical Directory, the Directory of American Specialists or other professional directory at your local library.

4

Drug Counselling, Mental Health and De-addiction

MENTAL HEALTH AND CHEMICAL DEPENDENCE SERVICES

New York's Partnership Plan programme includes a comprehensive and somewhat unique approach to the provision of mental health and alcohol and chemical dependence treatment services to enrolled beneficiaries. This study describes in some detail the programme that was implemented under the authority of the State's Section 1115 Waiver.

Identification of Mental Health and Chemical Dependence Needs

In accordance with the requirements outlined in the RFP and model contract, all MCOs must have policies and procedures to ensure that all network primary care providers routinely screen for mental health and substance abuse problems. The RFP and contract require MCOs to conduct a formalized health screening to assess for any special health (e.g., behavioural health services) needs that the member may have. The Department requires that the plans adopt practice guidelines consistent with current standards of care as recommended by the American Academy of Pediatrics, the U.S. Task Force on Preventive Care, the

New York State Child/Teen health Plan, New York State Prenatal Care Standards for Managed Care Plans, the US DHHS Center for Substance Abuse Treatment, and the AIDS Institute Clinical Standards for Adult and Pediatric Care. In addition, plans must have policies and procedures to ensure that members receive follow-up services from appropriate providers based on the findings of their assessment.

All MCOs must have policies and procedures to ensure that network and mental health providers appropriately evaluate the patient's treatment needs. NYS DOH encourages MCOs to train providers in the identification, implementation and use of validated assessment tools. MCOs must also have policies and procedures in place to ensure that members who have been evaluated and determined in need of treatment actually receive referrals to appropriate providers. As a part of the C/THP programme MCOs are also required to ensure that network providers appropriately screen children for behavioural and developmental problems and to make referrals for follow-up care and treatment as needed.

Finally, MCOs must have in place a mechanism through which high-risk patients can be evaluated and referred for treatment. This must include a referral mechanism whereby network primary care providers, including pediatricians, internists, family and general practitioners, obstetricians, and nurse practitioners may request that a MCO representative or behavioural health provider reach out to any patient they believe to be in need of mental health or chemical dependence treatment services and attempt to arrange for an evaluation of their needs.

The State requires that all mainstream MCOs report information on the utilisation of behavioural health care (mental health, chemical dependence) services, including inpatient and outpatient utilisation statistics, assessments of anti-depressant medication management and follow-up after hospitalisations for mental illness. The State Department of Health Office of Managed Care has identified indicators and is planning research studies to evaluate the provision of behavioural health care services for managed care enrollees. A description of these initiatives is included. This monitoring protocol focuses, among other things, on the number of complaints/grievances filed with MCOs or the state or counties (including New York City) regarding access to behavioural health care services by managed care enrollees. Mental Health Services for Persons with Serious and Persistent Mental Illness (SPMI) or Serious Emotional Disturbance (SED) (including persons dually diagnosed with Chemical Dependence problem)

Adults aged eighteen (18) and older who are diagnosed as seriously and persistently mentally ill and children through seventeen (17) years of age who are diagnosed as seriously emotionally disturbed qualify for a mental health exemption if they have utilized the following services during the twelve month period prior to scheduled enrollment:

- Ten (10) or more encounters, including visits to mental health clinic, psychiatrist or psychologist and inpatient hospital days relating to a psychiatric diagnosis; or
- One (1) or more specialty mental health visits (i.e., psychiatric rehabilitation treatment programme; day treatment; continuing day treatment; comprehensive case management; partial hospitalisation; rehabilitation services provided to residents of OMH licensed community residences and family-based treatment and mental health clinics for seriously emotionally disturbed children).

MCOs must permit all enrollees to self-refer to a network provider for an initial evaluation of a mental health problem without going through their primary care provider. MCOs must provide all medically necessary treatment in the least restrictive, clinically appropriate setting. Once a total MCO benefit of 20 outpatient visits or 30 inpatient days is reached, the State will reimburse plans for their reimbursable costs of providing services through a stop loss mechanism. Under the stop loss programme, the MCO will manage, coordinate and pay for mental health outpatient visits and inpatient hospital days for patients who exceed their 20 outpatient visits or 30 inpatient days benefit. The MCO will bill NYS Medicaid Programme for these services at the contracted fee schedule via the State's stop loss programme.

SSI SPMI/SED may enroll in health plans for a "health-only" benefit or remain fee-for-service. ADC/HR SPMI/SED persons may enroll for the same comprehensive health/ mental health benefit as other enrollees or may remain fee-for-service. To assure that all clients with serious mental illness are adequately informed about their enrollment options, the NYS DOH has sent out letters to all potential Medicaid managed care enrollees that address mental health exemptions. In addition, OMH and the department sent letters concerning the exemption option to providers of mental health services, local mental hygiene directors, local social service commissioners and consumer advocates. The letter provided information about the exemption process and medical documentation necessary to obtain an exemption. In addition, OMH staff routinely attend county Medicaid managed care implementation meetings.

Coordination of Service Delivery

Coordination between the Managed Care Plan and Out-of-Network Providers. Two distinct groups of managed care enrollees may, at any given point in time, receive behavioural health care services from out-of-network providers: SSI individuals with serious mental illness who are enrolled in the MCO for non-behavioural health care services only; and individuals who are receiving more intensive services which have been carved out of the capitated benefit package. In each case, managed care plans are expected to cooperate with these out-of-network providers to the extent reasonable, practical, and possible in ensuring that recipients receive care in a coordinated fashion. The State recognizes that individuals receiving care outside of the managed care plan may not always be forthcoming with their in-plan providers about the nature and extent of the treatment they are undergoing. All MCO enrollees will be encouraged to permit exchange of clinical information.

Persons with Chemical Dependency Problems

All persons requiring treatment for a chemical dependency problem who are members of one of the mandatory eligibility groups (in a local district approved for mandatory managed care enrollment must access such care through the mainstream MCO in which they are enrolled. MCOs must permit all enrollees to self-refer to a network provider for an initial chemical dependence assessment and evaluation for inpatient detoxification, inpatient rehabilitation or outpatient detoxification services without going through their primary care provider.

MCOs must provide all medically necessary treatment in the least restrictive, clinically appropriate setting. Once a total MCO benefit of 30 inpatient days for medically necessary and clinically appropriate Medicaid reimbursable inpatient chemical dependence rehabilitation and treatment is reached the State will reimburse plans for their reimbursable costs of providing services through a stop loss mechanism. There are no day limitations on inpatient detoxification when medically necessary (i.e., complicated DRGs) in an acute hospital setting. Inpatient and outpatient detoxification services do not count towards the behavioural health stop loss visit limits.

Under the stop loss programme, the MCO will manage, coordinate and pay for inpatient chemical dependence rehabilitation or treatment days for patients who exceed their 30 day inpatient benefit. The MCO will bill NYS Medicaid Programme for these services at the contracted fee schedule via the State's stop loss programme.

Welfare Reform related chemical dependency services requirements may be met regardless of whether the required services are provided as part of the Medicaid managed care capitated benefit package or reimbursed outside the benefit package. As of October 1, 2004, the contractor shall designate a Welfare Reform liaison who shall work with the LDSS or its designee to (1) ensure that enrollees receive timely access to assessments and services specified in the Medicaid managed care contract and (2) ensure completion of reports containing medical documentation required by the LDSS.

Persons requiring Mental Health Services who are Not Seriously and Persistently Mentally Ill or Emotionally Disturbed. Non-SPMI/SED persons who are required to enroll in managed care plans must obtain needed mental health services through their MCO. Managed care plans are required to provide all medically necessary mental health treatment services in the least restrictive, clinically appropriate setting and are at financial risk for the cost of services, up to the in-plan benefit limits imposed by the State. MCOs must permit enrollees to self-refer to a network behavioural health care provider for an initial assessment/ evaluation without going through their primary care provider.

MCOs must make available to their enrollees a complete listing of the behavioural health care providers in their network.

The capitated mental health benefit package provided by the HMOs and PHSPs includes up to 20 outpatient visits and 30 inpatient days (combined with chemical dependence). Specialized services, including Intensive Psychiatric Rehabilitation Treatment (IPRT), Continuing Day Treatment (CDT) for Adults and Day Treatment for Children, SED Clinic Services for Children, Intensive Case Management and Supportive Case Management (ICM/SCM), are not covered by the managed care plans. Individuals requiring these services will be referred to the local Department of Community Mental Health for assistance in obtaining this type of specialized care on a fee-for-service basis. Generally persons requiring this level of care will have been diagnosed with a serious mental illness, and the local district will need to counsel this individual about treatment options, including the option to disenroll from managed care if they so choose.

THE MENTAL HEALTH STATISTICS IMPROVEMENT PROGRAMME (MHSIP)

MHSIP began in 1976 as a collaboration between states and the National Institute of Mental Health to develop national data standards for use by state and local governments and individual mental health providers. The aim was to promote uniform collection and reporting of mental health statistical information through the voluntary adoption of data standards by mental health organisations. The first MHSIP product was <FN-8>, published in 1983. The concepts in that report were expanded and refined in 1989 with publication of <FN-10>, Data Standards for Mental Health Dec. Supp. Systems. Over the past twenty years several additional MHSIP reports have been produced about MH data, its uses and its users. MHSIP has grown so that its mission is now well beyond the task of producing only uniform standards for data collection. MHSIP now carries multiple meanings, including the following:

— MHSIP now represents a set of values centered around the commitment to the use of statistical information for decision support in the mental health service system, and in the inclusion of consumers and other stakeholders in aspects of system processes.

— MHSIP supports an evolving set of guidelines for best practices for the development of mental health data systems, including common definitions of terms and measures and reporting that are accessible to all stakeholders.

— MHSIP is supported, in part by, a Federal funding stream, that includes set-aside funds from the Mental Health Block Grant; the funds have been employed to assist states' efforts to improve their statistical systems and to initiate task forces that have produced data standards for MH data systems and best practice guidelines for performance indicator and report card development.

— Finally, MHSIP is an informal community of professionals, service recipients, and other advocates committed its goals.

Although MHSIP itself is just over 20 years old, it has roots that go back into the last century. The history of MHSIP is the history of federal reporting of mental health information, beginning with reporting on the numbers of persons in mental health institutions. These data were collected by the United States Census as far back as the 19 century. When the National Institute of Mental Health was established in 1946, federal efforts to maintain mental health data were incorporated into its functions. Today that responsibility rests with the Survey and Analysis Branch of the national Center for Mental Health Services, a part of the Substance Abuse and Mental Health Services Administration.

The direction of MHSIP is determined, in part, by an *ad hoc* group that meets several times each year to review and work on current projects, and to initiate new ones. Once limited to federal and state mental health officials, the committee membership has diversified to include recipients of mental health services, local providers of mental health services, staff of the National Association of State Mental Health Programme Directors, and officials of other federal agencies.

The MHSIP community meets annually at the National Conference on Mental Health Statistics, usually the week following Memorial Day Weekend. The National Conference—now in its 47th year—provides a forum for discussing major changes in federal and state policies and the direction of the public mental health system, as well as presentations of new ideas about best practices, workshops focussing on how to implement statistical methods, and reports on uses of mental health information.

Alternative Report Card Designs

Evaluation of mental health programmes has a long history, and the MHSIP Consumer-Oriented Mental Health Report Card, like others to be discussed below, borrows liberally from that literature and experience in its design. Programme evaluation efforts are typically limited to assessing outcomes for persons who are under treatment within a particular programme. What is conceptually different about the MHSIP Consumer-Oriented Mental Health Report

Card is that it is focussed, not on a particular person admitted to a particular programme, but on the population of persons enrolled in a managed care mental health plan, a plan which will necessarily include a range of programmes and services.

The first report card for a managed care plan was published by the Kaiser-Permanente Health Plan of Northern California in the early 1990s. It included two mental health performance indicators: rates of suicide for plan enrollees (in comparison to all persons residing in the same geographic area) and the rate at which persons receiving psychiatric inpatient care for major affective disorders had at least one outpatient visit within 30 days of discharge.

The first report card for a managed behavioural healthcare plan was published by United Behavioural Healthcare of Minneapolis. This report card had approximately a dozen indicators and was based upon data that the company already maintained in its management information system. This included the results of a client satisfaction survey undertaken on a sample of UBH enrollees who had received treatment. In addition to the MHSIP project, two prominent report cards were developed by the National Committee on Quality Assurance (NCQA) and the American Behavioural Healthcare Association (AMBHA). Each is briefly described below.

NCQA is a national organisation organised for the purpose of assessing the quality of care in health care plans. The board of the organisation is principally composed of representatives from health care plans and from the major employers who purchase services from them. Beginning in 1992, NCQA began pilot testing its Health Employee Data Information System (HEDIS), a system which required each health plan to produce indicators of plan performance.

The original HEDIS and successive versions have included a limited set of mental health indicators. Among those included were measures of penetration and utilisation for the categories of inpatient, ambulatory and day/night services. Rates were further broken down by age and gender groupings, as well as by payor/employer. Readmission rates for inpatient care were also incorporated. Subsequent versions of HEDIS have included a small number of additional indicators in a testing data set, and the addition of a satisfaction survey is also contemplated.

This survey may be based upon the MHSIP Consumer Survey or a survey under development as part of a larger health plan evaluation project, the Consumer Assessment of Health Plans Study (CAHPS). Specific HEDIS reporting requirements are issued each year, but changes to behavioural health indicators are typically made less frequently. In contrast to NCQA, AMBHA is an association of organisations that provide managed behavioural healthcare, not general healthcare (although some of its members are subsidiaries of organisations that offer managed healthcare).

Most of the largest such organisations are included in its membership. At the time that its report card project, PERMS, was undertaken, AMBHA members covered over 120 million lives for behavioural healthcare services. The PERMS project was announced by AMBHA in the fall of 1995, and data collection from its members proceeded over the next year. The plan was to produce an industry-wide performance report *without* identifying differences in performance among companies.

PERMS has a larger number of indicators. Like HEDIS, it includes utilisation rates, although breakdown categories include diagnosis and clinician type, as well as age, gender, and treatment setting; and rehospitalisation rates within

30 days with and without outpatient follow-up. In addition, PERMS includes expenditure rates by treatment settings, measures of telephone responsiveness, medication management visits for persons with a diagnosis of schizophrenia, and family visits for children under 12. Finally, PERMS incorporates six indicators based upon a consumer satisfaction survey. An updated version of the AMBHA PERMS, version 2.0, was released this summer.

There are several differences between the MHSIP, PERMS, and HEDIS report card designs.

— MHSIP is the most extensive with respect to mental health performance indicators. HEDIS and PERMS were both developed with the limitation that the indicators could be produced with little or no modification of existing data sets among member organisations. As noted earlier, the MHSIP design proceeded from a set of values articulated as formal goals and concerns within the public mental health system.

— The MHSIP design incorporates extensive outcome indicators, while the others do not; all three include indicators of access to and appropriateness of care.

— In the MHSIP design, consumer reports are the most important source of data. PERMS includes a few indicators based upon consumer reports. HEDIS is in the process of incorporating indicators based upon such measures.

— In the MHSIP design, the focus on persons who have serious mental illness is central; HEDIS and PERMS have few indicators that are appropriate for this population.

— The MHSIP design assumes a broad and flexible mental health benefit; in HEDIS and PERMS

> assumptions about what services are available to the insured population are unclear, but appear to be limited.

It has been assumed that the MHSIP design is the least feasible because it is the most extensive. In fact, both NCQA and AMBHA have experienced very significant problems in obtaining complete data from their member organisations. Despite the MHSIP Consumer-Oriented Mental Health Report Card's demands, it has gained relatively wide use in public mental health systems.

Design of the MHSIP Consumer-Oriented Mental Health Report Card

The MHSIP Policy Group initiated the report card project in the Fall of 1993 with funding support from the national Center for Mental Health Services (SAMHSA, PHS, USDHHS). Anticipating the development of a national managed care report card under the Administration's plan for healthcare reform, the Committee recognized a need to begin planning its mental health component. As events developed, the primary audience for the report card has been individual states proceeding in their own healthcare reform efforts. The first phase of work was the development of a conceptual definition of the report card. Under the leadership of John Hornik, a task force identified the major domains for evaluation of managed care plans providing mental health services. In May, 1994, at the National Conference on Mental Health Statistics, the task force presented the MHSIP community with a draft report for comment. With broad support the work proceeded into the next phase.

With new leadership in the person of Vijay Ganju, the Phase 2 task force proceeded to develop detailed operational definitions of performance indicators within each domain, including recommended measures and methods of data collection for each indicator. Like the first task force, this group included a wide array of participants including recipients of mental health services and family members, federal and state mental health and substance abuse officials, academic experts in services research, and providers of mental health services. Throughout its18 months of work, the task force formally and informally solicited the views of the groups from which its membership was drawn. At the May, 1996, annual conference, the MHSIP Consumer-Oriented Mental Health Report Card received an enthusiastic reception from the MHSIP community. In fact, several states had already begun to implement their own versions of the report card, based upon earlier drafts that had been circulated. The strengths of the design included the following:

1. Values. The report card is based upon a well-articulated set of values for the public mental health system. These are represented as specific "concerns" within each of the major report card domains (Access, Appropriateness, Outcomes, Health Promotion/Prevention). Each concern identifies a significant goal of mental health services (*e.g.,* Service recipients experience increased independent functioning). Twenty-six mental health plan goals provide the basis for rating performance; the largest number of goals (13) are in the outcomes domain.

2. Specificity. For each of the 26 concerns, there are between one and four performance indicators to assess how well the plan is performing in that goal area. Recommended measures are presented for each performance indicator. The measures include standardized instruments where the task force judged that these were appropriate and new measures in areas where there were no existing reliable measures.

3. Sources of Data. The design of the report card requires multiple sources of data to construct performance indicators. Most prominent among these is the report of service recipients themselves on their care and treatment outcomes. Clinician assessments, enrollment-encounter data, medical records, and plan financial information are also incorporated.

4. Population Sensitivity. The task force recognized the fact that different populations are served under managed care plans. While a primary focus was on assessing performance of plans serving persons with serious mental illness, the task force identified the subset of performance indicators that applied to other adults and children and to persons with substance abuse problems. It also identified specific performance indicators for children and adolescents with serious emotional disturbance.

Status of the MHSIP Consumer-Oriented Mental Health Report Card

The MHSIP Consumer-Oriented Mental Health Report Card has already had a wide influence upon state mental health authorities. In the wake of health care reform and the adoption of managed care approaches to public mental health services, approximately 30 states are in the process of adopting or adapting the MHSIP design in part or in whole. The most frequent adoption is of the MHSIP consumer survey, although it is not unusual for states to make local modifications or additions to this instrument. Fewer states have attempted to implement the indicators of the Report Card based on data other than the Consumer Survey. At least one state, New Mexico, did adopt the entire Report Card and did substantial work towards fine-tuning the non-survey indicators. Some states (*e.g.*, Delaware, New York) have also replicated the MHSIP Consumer-Oriented Mental Health Report Card development process, convening stakeholder groups for discussion of values and concerns in the public mental health system, as well as review of proposed performance indicators and measures.

How to Use This Toolkit

To date, the primary resource for MHSIP Consumer-Oriented Mental Health Report Card users has been the final Task Force report released in April 1996. While this document outlined the domains, indicators and measures necessary to implement the Report Card, the document did not provide guidance on a host of practical decisions that are required in implementing a performance measurement system. Because of this, a number of persons have turned to members of the MHSIP *ad hoc* Group and to the Evaluation Center@HSRI for technical assistance in implementing the Report Card. To avoid resource-intensive consultations to individuals, the MHSIP *ad hoc* Group agreed for the Evaluation Center@HSRI to develop a *Toolkit for Performance Measurement Using the MHSIP Consumer-Oriented Mental Health Report Card* that would provide guidance in a user-friendly, how-to format. The Evaluation Center has worked with a group of experts with experience implementing the Report Card to produce this first version of the *Toolkit*.

The Toolkit is organised into chapters based on major steps in Report Card implementation. While these major steps are presented in what is most often chronological order, we suggest that users read the entire Toolkit first, and then go back to focus on specific issues in turn. This will help you understand the overall dimensions of a Report Card project before getting bogged down in details. And, reading about steps that occur later in the process may affect your thinking in the early stages.

Wherever possible, we have built on the concrete experience of persons who have implemented the Report Card. In addition, we have tried to identify resources for more detailed information on topics that we address only briefly. This study includes a number of recommendations. These recommendations represent the thinking of one or more of the contributors, and in many cases reflect a group discussion and consensus. For quick reference, we have pulled out the major recommendations within each chapter and displayed these at the close of the study.

TREATMENT PHILOSOPHY: AN INTRODUCTION

Cocaine abuse and addiction represent a significant health problem in the United States (NIDA 1994). In recent years, this problem has increased, inflicting much harm on addicted individuals, their families, and society. Many individuals with cocaine problems have other substance use disorders, medical problems, psychiatric disorders, and psychosocial problems.

Cocaine is taken by mouth, inhaled, injected into the veins, and smoked. In recent years, the number of cocaine users who smoke crack cocaine has increased. Cocaine stimulates the central nervous system (CNS) to produce an increase in energy and psychomotor activity; a heightened sense of sensory arousal, pleasure, and euphoria; and a decrease in appetite and the need for sleep. It affects judgment and behaviour, as well. Physical, behavioural, and social problems are common among cocaine addicts and may include any of the following specific consequences (Weaver and Schnoll 1999, pp. 105-120):

— *Physical:* Cardiovascular (for example, hypertension, arrhythmia, cardiomyopathy, myocarditis, myocardial ischemia, myocardial infarction), head and neck (erosion of dental enamel, rhinitis, perforation of nasal septum), CNS (headache, seizures), lung damage, pneumonia, chronic cough, acute renal failure, sexual dysfunction, spontaneous abortion in pregnant women, and infections (HIV, hepatitis B or C, tetanus) from sharing needles.

— *Psychological:* Poor judgment, anxiety, depression, suicidal feelings and behaviours, insomnia, emotional instability, irritability, aggressive behaviour, and psychotic symptoms. Symptoms of psychiatric disorders such as schizophrenia, panic disorder, depression, or mania can be triggered or exacerbated by cocaine use or withdrawal.

— *Social/family:* Damaged or lost relationships, child abuse or neglect, lost jobs, accidents, prostitution, spread of infections, criminal behaviours, violent behaviours, and homicide.

As a result of the significant health and social problems caused by cocaine abuse and addiction, the National Institute on Drug Abuse (NIDA) has sponsored a number of studies of different cocaine treatment approaches. This Group Drug Counselling (GDC) manual describes one of the psychosocial treatments developed for use in a multisite clinical trial called the Collaborative Cocaine Treatment Study (CCTS). The study was conducted at Brookside Hospital in Nashua, New Hampshire, the University of Pennsylvania in Philadelphia, the University of Pittsburgh Medical Center (Western Psychiatric Institute and Clinic) in Pittsburgh, and Harvard Medical School (McLean Hospital in Belmont, Massachusetts, and Massachusetts General Hospital in Boston) (Crits-Christoph et al. 1997, pp. 721-726). All study sites randomly assigned cocaine dependent clients to one of four treatment conditions:

— Individual Drug Counselling (IDC) with GDC (Mercer and Woody 2000).

— Individual Supportive-Expressive Psychotherapy

(SEP) with GDC (Luborsky 1984).

— Individual Cognitive Therapy (CT) with GDC (Beck et al. 1993).

— GDC alone.

Each of the three individual treatments, IDC, SEP, and CT, and the GDC treatment were described in manuals that guided the clinical approach used with clients. All study therapists participated in intensive training and ongoing supervision during the course of the pilot study and the main clinical trial, and their work was taped and independently rated to ensure that they adhered to the specific model of treatment they were using. IDC, SEP, and CT involved 6 months of active treatment. During the first 3 months of treatment, counsellors offered clients individual sessions twice a week. During months four through six, counsellors offered clients individual treatment sessions once a week. Clients were offered monthly booster sessions during months seven through nine. Clients could select a total of 39 individual therapy sessions while they participated in the treatment protocol. In addition, all clients assigned to the three individual treatment groups were offered GDC sessions weekly for 24 sessions: 12 weekly sessions in a structured psychoeducational group and 12 weekly sessions in an unstructured problemsolving group. Thus, clients assigned to any of the three individual treatments could attend up to 63 individual and group sessions during the study. One of every four clients was randomly assigned to GDC alone, and short case management sessions were available to them as needed. These clients primarily participated in group sessions and were offered 24 sessions during a 6-month period, followed by monthly individual case management sessions during months seven through nine.

Adaptation of the GDC Model to Community Programmes

Although the research study found that all treatments helped patients improve, the combination of IDC and GDC produced the best results (Crits-Christoph et al. 1999, pp. 493-502). Community addiction outpatient treatment programmes may not be able to offer as many treatment sessions as were offered in the treatment research study due to constraints imposed by managed care and changes in funding substance abuse services. Even with limited sessions, an IDC + GDC treatment model can be offered. For example, if a client is approved for 20 outpatient sessions, 12 could be offered as group sessions and 8 as individual sessions. While group sessions can be provided weekly, individual sessions can be spread out every several weeks or more so that patients stay connected to treatment for at least 3 months. Evidence shows that drug abusers need a minimum of 3 months in outpatient treatment to benefit from treatment (Simpson et al. 1997). Because keeping clients in treatment for 3 months or longer is important, clinicians should use multiple strategies to improve treatment adherence (Daley and Zuckoff 1999; Carroll 1998; Blackwell 1976; Meichenbaum and Turk 1987; Daley et al. 1998).

Development of the GDC Model

The GDC approach was developed based on extensive clinical experience conducting addiction recovery groups and on a review of the relevant literature. Group therapy is one of the primary approaches used to treat drug addiction, including cocaine dependence (Rawson et al. 1989; Washton 1989; McAuliffe and Albert 1992; Vannicelli 1995; Washton 1997; Khantzian et al. 1999). Treatment groups are used throughout the continuum of care, from inpatient to intensive out-patient to aftercare programmes. Clients often complain that addiction treatment that is provided only in groups is too limited, and many want individual as well as group sessions. Experience in this study as well as in clinical work supports the notion that a combination of individual and group treatment for cocaine addiction is preferable.

The GDC model addresses common issues in the early and middle stages of recovery from addiction. The philosophy of the GDC approach is that cocaine addiction, and other chemical addictions are complex biopsychosocial diseases that are often chronic and debilitating. Many biological, psychological, sociocultural, and spiritual factors interact to contribute to the development and maintenance of cocaine and other types of substance addictions (Daley and Marlatt 1997).

Addiction causes or exacerbates a variety of biopsychosocial problems in the addicted person as well as in the family. Adverse consequences associated with addiction include medical diseases, psychological and psychiatric disorders, family and interpersonal problems, and legal, economic, occupational, academic, and spiritual problems (Weiss and Mirin 1995; Earley 1991).

Participation in Self-Help Programmes

The GDC model strongly encourages participation in 12-Step self-help recovery programmes such as Cocaine Anonymous (CA), Narcotics Anonymous (NA), and Alcoholics Anonymous (AA). The importance of actively participating in these programmes is emphasized in group sessions. Talking at meetings, learning and using the 12 Steps, using slogans, socializing before and after meetings, calling other members, and relating to a sponsor are ways clients can actively participate in the fellowship. Analysis of data from the CCTS showed that clients who actively participated in self-help activities had better outcomes than those who attended meetings without actively participating (Weiss 1996).

Symptoms of Addiction

Although each client may evidence a unique pattern of cocaine addiction, he or she will manifest three or more of the symptoms listed below. These are based on the following criteria for substance dependency from DSM-IV of the American Psychiatric Association's Diagnostic and Statistical Manual of Mental Disorders (American Psychiatric Association 1994, pp. 175-272).

- Excessive or inappropriate use of cocaine (or other substances): For example, getting high on cocaine or other drugs or getting drunk on alcohol and not being able to fulfill obligations at home, at work, or with others; feeling as if cocaine or other substances are needed to fit in with others or function at work or at home; or driving under the influence of substances.
- Preoccupation with getting or using chemicals: For example, living mainly to get high on cocaine, other drugs, and/or alcohol; making substance use too important in life; or being obsessed with using cocaine or other substances.
- Change in one's tolerance for addictive substances: For example, needing more cocaine or other substances to get high or getting high much more easily and by using less of the substance than was used in the past.
- Having trouble reducing or abstaining from cocaine or other substance use: For example, not being able to control how much or how often one uses cocaine or other substances or using more cocaine or other substances than planned.
- Withdrawal symptoms: For example, getting sick physically, including having the shakes, feeling

nauseous, having gooseflesh, having a runny nose, etc., once one cuts down or stops using cocaine or other substances; or experiencing mental symptoms such as depression, anxiety, or agitation.

— Using cocaine and other substances to avoid or stop withdrawal symptoms: For example, using cocaine or other substances to prevent withdrawal sickness or drinking or using drugs to stop withdrawal symptoms once they've started.

— Using cocaine or other substances even though they cause problems in one's life: For example, not taking a doctor's, therapist's, or other professional's advice to stop using because of problems substances have caused in one's life.

— Giving up important activities or losing friendships because of cocaine or other substance use: For example, discontinuing participation in activities that once were important, giving up friends who don't get high, losing friends because of how cocaine or other substance use affects relationships with others.

— Stopping cocaine or other substance use for a period of time (days, weeks, or months), only to begin again: For example, promising to quit using cocaine or other substances only to begin getting high again or being unable to remain abstinent from cocaine or other drugs.

— Getting into trouble because of cocaine or other substance use: For example, losing jobs or being unable to find a job, getting arrested or having other legal problems; sabotaging relationships or having trouble with family or friends, or having money problems because of cocaine or other substance use.

Because cocaine addiction is a disease that involves losing control of cocaine and other substance use, addicted individuals often enter treatment feeling demoralized and out of control. They enter a treatment programme to help them regain control of their lives. Thus, treatment must provide a safe, structured environment through regular, frequent contact with the treatment staff.

Abstinence from all drugs is the primary goal of treatment in the treatment protocol. Changing one's lifestyle, solving problems, and improving coping skills are additional goals that help support the overall goal of abstaining from cocaine or other substances.

STABILISATION PROCEDURES

The first step in treating cocaine addiction is detoxifying the client from cocaine and other addictive drugs. Immediately upon entering treatment, the client participates in a brief stabilisation phase designed to detoxify him or her from addictive drugs, to assess psychosocial stability, and/or to begin to establish basic recovery supports. The group counsellor works with the client throughout the stabilisation period.

The goals of the stabilisation phase of treatment are to:

- Help the client establish abstinence from cocaine and other drugs.
- Help the client become motivated to participate in ongoing treatment sessions.
- Assess the client's psychosocial stability, i.e., whether he or she lacks a stable, drug-free living environment or has significant psychopathology that may interfere with his or her benefiting from the cocaine recovery programme.

— Provide education and support to help the client increase his or her knowledge of cocaine addiction and recovery and encourage him or her to engage in treatment and the recovery processes.

This phase of treatment lasts up to 2 weeks. Some clients complete detoxification from cocaine use before they start group treatment. Others continue to use cocaine or other substances even though they have started treatment. In such cases, treatment aims to help them focus on strategies to initiate abstinence. Not all clients begin the treatment programme with the same level of motivation or become substance free before attending actual treatment sessions.

Brief, frequent contact with a counsellor is helpful for the cocaine addict attempting to detoxify and stabilize on an outpatient basis. Of course, some clients with severe addiction problems are best detoxified in a hospital or addiction rehabilitation programme and may enter outpatient treatment following an inpatient stay. Others enter outpatient treatment after completing a brief residential addiction programme. During the detoxification and stabilisation phase, the group counsellor sees the client 2 to 5 days each week. Clients typically attend treatment sessions two to three times a week. Clients may attend as many as five sessions of treatment a week if they are detoxifying from alcohol or another substance in addition to cocaine, or if they express a need for additional support. Each stabilisation visit lasts 10 to 30 minutes.

Drug Testing

Drug testing with urinalysis and Breathalyzer is an important component of the treatment programme. Frequent drug testing helps support the client's abstinence by holding that person accountable for his or her behaviour. Accountability, responsibility, and honesty must be consistently fostered in recovery because these values are often displaced by one's addictive behaviour. Therefore, the addicted person benefits from reclaiming these values in recovery.

Throughout treatment, clients' urine is screened routinely for the presence of drugs. The group counsellor collects the urine at the group sessions. For the first 2 months of treatment, following stabilisation, clients' urine is collected twice a week. During the 3rd through 6th month of treatment, the clients' urine is collected for analysis once a week, at the group sessions. Breathalyzer data is collected on the same schedule used to collect the urine.

Results of urinalyses are returned to the group counsellor. When a client's urine tests positive for cocaine or other drugs, the group counsellor is responsible for discussing this information with the client individually. Clients are strongly encouraged to discuss any cocaine or other drug use in their group sessions. However, it is the client's decision whether to disclose his or her drug use to the group, although disclosing this information is encouraged.

Focus of Stabilisation Visits

The stabilisation visits focus on:

- Monitoring and discussing any cocaine or other substance use, cravings, or close calls to use with the client.
- Educating the client about the detoxification process, including the physical and psychological symptoms that may be experienced during withdrawal. The counsellor monitors withdrawal symptoms and teaches the client about cocaine-related medical problems and other types of substance use disorders.
- Helping the client identify the people, places, and

things that can trigger cocaine cravings, and encouraging the client to find ways to avoid these triggers or cope with them without using addictive substances.

— Encouraging the client to participate in self-help programmes such as AA, CA, or NA, or other self-help groups. The counsellor provides the client with information about different types of meetings of these programmes, the location of meetings, etc. The counsellor answers the client's questions about the philosophy of 12-step programmes and other self-help programmes that might be available to the client. Any concerns the client has about participating in a self-help programme are discussed.

— Conducting Breathalyzer testing and urinalysis at each visit during the stabilisation phase of treatment.

— Referring the client to needed ancillary services such as medical care, welfare, food stamps, vocational assistance, and stable living arrangements.

OVERVIEW OF GROUP TREATMENT FOR COCAINE ADDICTION

Group treatment sessions are a vital aspect of recovery from cocaine addiction. Groups give clients the opportunity to learn the facts about cocaine addiction and recovery so that they can better understand their drug use problems. Clients also gain strength and hope from each other, learn to use and benefit from social support, and begin to feel valued because they are helping others who are trying to recover from cocaine addiction. Although specific group sessions vary in content and focus during Phase I (weeks 1-12) and II (weeks 13-24), the general purpose of group treatment is to provide members with an opportunity to:

— *Acquire information* about important concepts and aspects of recovery from addiction to cocaine or other substances. This includes but is not limited to information on:
  - Symptoms of addiction dependence and withdrawal
  - Factors contributing to addiction
  - The recovery process
  - Biopsychosocial issues in recovery
  - Phases of recovery and common problems experienced in each phase
  - Cocaine and other drug cravings
  - Social pressures to use substances
  - People, places, events, and things that trigger substance use
  - Effects of cocaine addiction on family and other relationships
  - Self-help groups
  - Support systems
  - How to cope with feelings
  - Guilt and shame
  - Relapse risk factors
  - Relapse warning signs
  - Tools for use in ongoing recovery

— *Become more aware* of their own problems and issues and how they relate to cocaine addiction and recovery. The group counsellor encourages clients to relate personally to the material presented or discussed in sessions.

— *Give support* to and *receive support* from each other by providing feedback and sharing problems, successes, hopes, and strength. Through the group experience, group members learn the importance of mutual support. They also learn the importance of confronting negative attitudes and managing unhealthy behaviours.

— *Learn recovery coping skills* to deal with problems that contribute to or result from the addiction, to reduce the chances of a relapse to cocaine addiction and to improve functioning. These coping skills include cognitive, behavioural, and interpersonal skills that can be used to manage the various challenges of recovery.

Content and Process of Groups

Roles of the Counsellor and Interventions

Group counsellors function as educators and counsellors, and they use a variety of interventions to conduct group sessions in both phases of treatment. These interventions include:

— Providing information about addiction and recovery and clarifying issues and answering questions related to the content of the sessions, particularly in Phase I.

— Helping members relate personally to the psychoeducational concepts discussed. The group counsellor tries to get members to relate less intellectually and more personally to the material.

— Facilitating group interaction among clients so that all members participate and share their thoughts, feelings, and experiences.

— Validating issues or struggles presented by individual

members. If a group member is struggling with relapse, the group counsellor acknowledges the struggle without being judgmental and tries to elicit support from other members of the group.

— Modeling healthy behaviours. This may involve providing positive reinforcement or modeling healthy communication with others.

— Challenging counterproductive activities and behaviours. This may involve giving a group member feedback on his or her current behaviour and pointing out behaviours that interfere with the group's ability to achieve its goals.

— Monitoring drug use or "close calls." The group counsellor structures group sessions to discuss episodes of substance use as well as strong cravings or close calls. Members can learn a lot from each other's mistakes.

— Encouraging attendance at self-help groups, particularly 12-step groups. This therapy model supports a positive view of AA, NA, and CA programmes. However, it is recognized that some group members won't attend 12-step meetings but may benefit from other types of self-help programmes.

— Motivating members to talk directly to each other when sharing their opinions, discussing experiences, or providing feedback. The group counsellor should be less of an "expert" and more of a facilitator during discussions of recovery concerns, problems, and issues.

Group counsellors should encourage all members of the group to participate in every session by voicing their opinions, feelings, and experiences as they relate to the topic covered. Group counsellors should draw quiet members into the discussion by asking them direct questions or seeking their opinions (e.g., "John, what is your experience with the issue of denial?" or "Madge, how do you relate to what's been discussed about relapse warning signs?"). Group counsellors should not let a member dominate the group discussions and should set limits as needed (e.g., "Carlton, I appreciate the fact that you have a lot of ideas to offer the group. Let's hear from some other members now to see how they relate to...." or "Lisa, it's great you have so many experiences or ideas to share, but we want to make sure others get a chance to talk, too.").

Group counsellors should provide positive reinforcement to both the group and individual members to foster group cohesion and trust. Reinforcement should be given even when a member talks about a lapse or relapse (e.g., "Luwanda, it's good that you talked to the group about your recent relapse and asked for their input.").

A key component of group sessions is realistic feedback about members' attitudes or behaviours. When possible, the group counsellor should encourage group members to provide feedback to another member who shows negative attitudes or behaviours (e.g., "Mike, what do you think about Jack's statement that NA meetings are a waste of time?" or "Liz, what do you think about Jack's statement that a few beers or joints won't hurt, that as long as he stays clean from cocaine he'll be OK?"). Similarly, positive feedback can be elicited from group members to support efforts made by another member (e.g., "What do others think about how Fran was able to resist her strong urge to smoke crack?").

The group counsellor also can provide direct feedback to an individual client or to the group by simply commenting on what he or she has observed. This type of intervention serves as a "model" for the other group members to use to provide feedback. It also provides members of the group with an opportunity to hear the group counsellor's perspective on an individual member (e.g., "John, I notice that when other members give you feedback, you interrupt them or argue with them." or "Mary, you did a great job talking about how your addiction really messed up your life. It takes a lot of courage to be so honest.") or on the group ("I notice that the discussion has shifted away from the topic of relationships in recovery to...." or "Your group did a nice job today talking about the ways AA and NA can aid recovery."). At times, a group member is in a state of crisis because he or she has suffered a recent lapse or relapse. The group counsellor can enlist some group members to help this member explore the lapse/relapse so that he or she may learn from it and develop a way to stop it. Other life problems may create crises for some group members, as well. Although the group counsellor can adhere to the principle of "disturbance takes precedence," in Phase I, the group counsellor must guard against spending too much time helping individual members resolve specific crises at the expense of reviewing the psychoeducational material pertaining to recovery. The group leader can see a member with a serious crisis before or after the group meets or during a scheduled appointment the next day. This member also can be encouraged to discuss the current crisis with an AA/NA/CA sponsor or with friends.

Client Orientation to Group Treatment

The group counsellor meets with each client before starting Phase I or II group sessions. During this orientation session, the counsellor discusses how important recovery groups are in the addiction treatment programme. Participating in recovery groups can help clients establish and maintain abstinence by providing additional structure and "positive peer pressure" to encourage them to follow through with recovery-oriented activities. Clients are told that they will learn important information about addiction and recovery and begin to develop coping skills to aid their recovery. The group provides supportive contact with caring, well-trained counsellors as well as with peers who are working on their own recovery. The counsellor also informs the client about the logistics of the group sessions and reviews the focus of Phase I and II.

Group rules also are reviewed during the orientation, and the client signs a form agreeing to abide by these rules. The rules encourage clients to come to group sessions free of the influence of cocaine or other substances, make a commitment to attend weekly group meetings, call to explain why he or she was absent from any group meetings, discuss close calls or actual episodes of cocaine or other substance use, and maintain confidentiality.

Phases of Group Treatment

In this GDC model, group treatment for cocaine addiction is provided in two phases. These phases coincide approximately with clients' needs in recovery, although individuals in recovery progress at their own pace. Clients are expected to begin Phase I as soon as they start the stabilisation phase of treatment. Starting in groups right away provides them with group support in the early phase of recovery and helps them in their efforts to initiate abstinence.

The treatment groups have a rolling admissions policy. That is, a client may enter the group at any session because a single recovery topic is covered completely within each session during Phase I. The counsellor tries to make each recovery topic equally beneficial for all clients, regardless of what stage of recovery they are in.

Phase I of the group treatment involves the first 12 weeks of therapy and is structured and psychoeducational in nature. Each Phase I session uses a curriculum with specific objectives that relate to an important aspect of addiction and recovery. Phase I provides an overview of the key issues in early recovery related to addiction, the recovery process, and relapse prevention.

PROBLEM-SOLVING GROUP

Following completion of Phase I group (weeks 1-12), clients participate in Phase II group during weeks 13 through 24. Phase II of the group treatment programme is a semi-structured, problem-solving session that meets for 12 consecutive weekly sessions of 90 minutes duration. By the time they enter Phase II, many clients have established some stability in their abstinence from cocaine and other substances. They have to continue actively working at staying sober and making positive changes in themselves and their lifestyle. Problem-oriented discussions provide group members with a context in which they take responsibility for addressing current problems, figure out coping strategies, receive ideas from other members regarding problems, and receive feedback from the group regarding their attitude or approach to dealing with life problems or ongoing recovery. Giving and receiving help and support also teaches group members the importance of self-disclosure, trust, and reciprocity.

The goals of Phase II group sessions are to help members:

— Identify and prioritize current problems in their daily lives that result from their cocaine addiction or potentially contribute to relapse risk, if not addressed.

— Develop strategies to cope with problems that are identified as increasing their chances of staying drug free and functioning better.
— Identify recovery issues or areas of change and strategies to address these.
— Give and receive support and feedback from each other regarding their recovery and how they cope with current problems.
— Address lapse and relapse crises and strategies to return to abstinence.
— Learn the process of problem-solving and how it can be applied to different problems in recovery or life.

Group Counsellor's Roles

In the problem-solving group, the group counsellor's main role is to facilitate the identification of problems in recovery and the discussion of strategies to address these problems. In the course of the group sessions, the group counsellor can educate; stimulate members to talk with each other rather than with the group counsellor; help members clarify and explore problems, concerns, and coping strategies; and help members support and confront one another. The group counsellor also protects the group process by ensuring that a balance exists among the three components of group treatment: 1) the "I" (individual group member); 2) the "we" (group as a unit or system); and 3) the "it" (problems or issues discussed). To help the group function, the group counsellor addresses problems that disrupt the group process, such as a member dominating the discussions, members failing to listen to each other, or members avoiding confronting unhealthy behaviours.

Group Format

1. Members are encouraged to socialize informally prior

to the start of the Phase II group session, while the group counsellor collects urine samples and has members take an alcohol Breathalyzer test.

2. The group formally starts with each member stating his name, admitting to the addiction, and providing the last date of cocaine or other substance use. During this "check-in" period, members are also encouraged to provide a brief update on their lives during the past week and discuss strong cravings or close calls regarding cocaine or other substance use.

3. Group members who have lapsed or relapsed since last session will briefly discuss the event in terms of warning signs and contributing factors. They will also be encouraged to develop a plan to return to abstinence and prevent future relapses.

4. At times, the focus of the entire group session may evolve from current struggles of group members to stay clean from drugs. Other times, the check-in period takes between 10 to 25 minutes.

5. Following the check-in period, each member states a current problem or concern in his life.

6. Once each group member has identified a problem or concern, the group begins to prioritize and discuss one or more of these issues. Often, problems and concerns discussed will overlap. Even if all group members do not get a chance to discuss their own problems, they can benefit from the process of mutual problem-solving within the group. Learning problem-solving skills that they can apply to recovery or life problems is one of the main goals of Phase II group sessions.

7. During the course of the discussions of a specific

problem, group members are encouraged to relate personally to the problem or issue discussed. They are asked to share their ideas on causes and effects of the problem and to give feedback to the member(s) presenting the problem. Feedback may relate to giving ideas on coping strategies or challenging the member's attitudes or behaviours in relation to the problem presented. The problem-solving component of these group sessions takes about 1 hour.

8. When about 10 to 15 minutes are left in the group session, the group counsellor reminds the group of the amount of time left and wraps up the discussion. During the final 10 to 15 minutes, each group member briefly summarizes one thing he or she learned from the group discussion and/or steps he or she plans to take during the upcoming week to aid his or her recovery from cocaine addiction.

9. The group ends with members joining hands and reciting the Serenity Prayer out loud.

Problems Encountered in the Group Process

In addition to specific problems related to recovery or the lives of the group members, problems are also commonly encountered in the group process. These problems require the group counsellor to intervene to make sure the group addresses them. Following is a discussion of some of the more common group process problems and suggested strategies for the group counsellor to undertake:

1. A group member dominates the discussion or always brings the discussion back to his own problems or issues. The group counsellor can thank the member for the contributions and then elicit opinions and experiences from other group members. If the group member persistently tries to dominate group discussions or always turns the

discussion back to his own problems or issues, this behaviour pattern can be pointed out by the group counsellor to make this member and other group members aware of the behaviour. The other members can be asked how they feel about the member's dominating the discussion, and how they want to deal with this in a way that is satisfying to everyone in the group. Even though this creates a problem on one level, on another level some group members find that it creates a safety net for them because they may believe they don't have to disclose personal problems or feelings as long as another member is taking up the group time.

2. A member does not disclose any problem or open up in the group session. The group counsellor can share his observations about the member's behaviour and generalize the issues by asking group members to talk about difficulties that contribute to problems in self-disclosing (e.g., shame, shyness, social anxiety). Discussion can then focus on ways this member (or other group members who have trouble disclosing) can gradually learn to trust the group to disclose personal thoughts, feelings, problems, or concerns.

3. A member consistently rejects the input, advice, or feedback of other group members. The group counsellor can point out this pattern and engage the group in a discussion of why this pattern is occurring. Members who offer help and support only to have their attempts rejected can be asked to talk about what this feels like so that the member who rejects their help is aware of the impact this behaviour has on others.

4. A member can only pay attention when the discussion focuses on his problems, or he interrupts others when they talk. The group counsellor can point out what he observes about the group member and discuss the reasons for this

behaviour. The group can then discuss the effects of this behaviour (e.g., upsets other members, turns them off, makes them feel as if their problems aren't important). The group can also discuss the importance of "giving and receiving" mutual support by listening to each other's concerns and problems.

5. A member wants easy answers to problems or is quick to provide easy solutions to others when they discuss personal problems. The group counsellor can share his observations of the behavioural patterns of this group member and ask the group to discuss the importance of taking responsibility for finding solutions to their problems and to identify more than one strategy to address a particular problem. The leader can emphasize that while there are many different ways to resolve specific problems, seldom are there easy or simple solutions, and that group members need time, patience, and persistence to adequately resolve problems. When a group member provides an easy solution, the group counsellor can acknowledge that this is one strategy that may help some people, but it is also helpful to have other strategies. The group counsellor can then engage the group in a discussion of other strategies to address the problem under discussion. Finally, the group counsellor can emphasize that learning how to think about problem solving is just as important as dealing with specific problems because everyone in the group will continue to face problems in his or her ongoing recovery.

6. A member tries to engage the group counsellor in individual therapy during the group session. The group counsellor can ask other group members to comment on the problems or issues this member presents. If the group member asks the group counsellor how to handle a specific problem, the counsellor first can encourage the member to identify

possible coping strategies, then ask other group members for their ideas for dealing with the problem.

7. A member arrives late for the group session or wants to leave during discussions. The leader and group members should develop a rule about arriving late for group sessions. Sometimes, there are legitimate reasons for being late (e.g., the bus a member takes was running 15 minutes late, the member got a flat tire, etc.). Members may be given a break once or twice for being late. However, the group may establish a rule that states that a member cannot join the group after a certain time (e.g., more than 10 minutes after the start of the group session). If time limits are not set, the group counsellor can predict that some members will be late often. Members who are persistently late can be asked to discuss this pattern of behaviour, how it is repeated in other areas of their lives, and what they think needs to be done to change this pattern. Group members should never leave a counselling session unless there is an emergency (e.g., they have a minor illness and need to use the restroom). Routinely allowing people to walk in and out disrupts the flow of the conversation and gives the message that what members say is not important. Members may want to leave group sessions because they are bored, feel like the discussions don't relate to them, or want to avoid discussing their own problems or concerns.

8. The group talks in generalities and avoids exploring specific problems in depth. The group counsellor can point out this dynamic to the group and ask members to discuss why they aren't talking about specific problems or concerns in recovery. The counsellor can ask members to set the agenda in a concrete way so that specific problems or concerns are identified for discussion. It isn't uncommon for group members to view counselling groups as no different than

free floating discussions held in some CA, NA, or AA meetings. However, Phase II group sessions are designed to explore and address problems and not simply be a repetition of 12-Step recovery meetings.

9. The group avoids confronting a member who behaves inappropriately. The group counsellor can point out this dynamic and ask group members what they think about the inappropriate behaviour and why they have avoided discussing it. Other problems may occur during the group time, but those described above are some of the more commonly occurring ones. While the "content" (i.e., problems and issues discussed) of the group is important, if the "process" bogs down, not much will be accomplished. In addition, some group members may miss sessions or drop out as a result of group process problems that aren't addressed. Unfortunately, group members may avoid bringing up the issues so the group counsellor won't always know the reasons for a member's poor attendance or early drop out from the group. It is not uncommon for members to be upset over process issues. A "preventive" strategy is to periodically engage the group in a discussion of the group process. The group counsellor can ask what members think about the group sessions, what they like and dislike about how the group has been going, and what changes they would like to see occur in the group.

Reasons for Dropping Out of Group Treatment

One of the assessments used in the CCTS study was called "Reasons for Early Termination of Treatment." This assessment aimed to find out specific reasons why clients left outpatient treatment before completing it. While clients gave numerous reasons for dropping out of the individual and group treatment conditions, the most common reasons they gave for dropping out of group treatment were:

— Time problems 42.7%
— Using cocaine again or wanting to use cocaine 30.7%
— Group sessions not helpful 30.7%
— Want a different treatment (individual) 30.7%
— Problems improved 18.7%
— Other unspecified reasons 18.7%
— Unwilling to participate in treatment 16.0%
— Needed hospitalisation 13.3%

Clients who participated in group treatment were more likely to find that group sessions alone were not as helpful as group sessions combined with IDC, CT, or Supportive Expressive therapy. This reinforces the point that clients generally do not like to participate in group-only treatment. They both want and need individual sessions, so a combination treatment is preferable when possible.

Common Issues or Problems Discussed in Phase II Group Sessions

Any of the recovery issues discussed in Phase I sessions may be revisited in Phase II problem-solving sessions. The most common issues discussed are those related to staying away from cocaine use, using other substances such as marijuana or alcohol, relapse, relationships, and making positive changes in oneself or one's lifestyle. Specific problems and issues discussed in groups include:

1. Motivational struggles: These include struggles such as loss of or diminished desire to stay drug free or to make personal and lifestyle changes. Motivational problems are reflected in a denial or minimisation of one's addiction to cocaine, lack of acceptance of the addiction, and failure to accept the need for abstinence as the goal of treatment. Motivational problems often lead to poor attendance at

treatment sessions, self-help groups, or lack of compliance with the individualized recovery plan. Poor attendance and compliance, in turn, often contribute to substance use relapse.

2. Strong desires, obsessions, or craving to use cocaine or other substances: These are more common among members who have not established any significant period of continuous abstinence from cocaine or other drugs. For members who have established continuous abstinence, significant increases in cravings or obsessions may occur in response to stress or problems. These strong desires also may indicate a risk of relapsing.

3. Lapse or relapse to cocaine or other drug use: Group members vary widely in their experiences with lapses or relapses. Some have none, others have one, and still others have multiple relapses during the course of treatment. Clients are not discharged for not achieving or maintaining abstinence. Instead, the focus is on trying to get each group member to develop a desire to initiate and maintain abstinence. It is expected that all positive urinalysis test results members have will be discussed in the Phase II group session. Clients can be referred to higher levels of care to re-establish stability if relapses are severe and the client simply cannot stop on his or her own.

4. Using other substances such as alcohol or marijuana: Some members have a strong desire to give up cocaine, the main drug of abuse, but continue using marijuana or alcohol. Although total abstinence is the main goal of treatment, some members will not accept this and may continue to use these other substances. While use of the substances increases the risk of cocaine relapse, the reality is that some group members will be able to limit their use of the other substances, particularly alcohol. However, the GDC model encourages total abstinence. The group counsellor facilitates discussion

of the potential risks of using other substances and asks group members who have tried unsuccessfully to do this in the past to share their experiences with the member who wishes to continue using other substances.

5. Problems related to participation in NA, CA, and AA or other self-help groups: Members vary in their use of self-help groups such as NA, CA, or AA. While attendance and active participation are highly encouraged, some clients refuse to attend, attend only occasionally, or participate minimally in the nuts and bolts of the programmes, such as getting a sponsor, working the steps, or attending social functions sponsored by NA, CA, or AA. Some members discuss problems such as conflicts with a sponsor or other members.

6. Relationship problems with family members, friends, or colleagues at work: Interpersonal problems run the gamut from mildly distressing ones to severe ones that pose a major threat to recovery or well being. Some specific interpersonal problems or issues discussed include conflicts or disputes with others, anger at or disappointment in others, emotional or physical violence, inappropriate sexual interactions (e.g., unprotected sex, sex with a stranger, sexual promiscuity), involvement in relationships that are nonsupportive or characterized by lack of reciprocity, difficulty saying no or setting limits with others, and difficulty asking others for help or support.

7. Upsetting emotional states such as persistent anxiety, boredom, depression, loneliness, guilt, or shame: The use of cocaine or other substances offers an immediate escape or relief from unpleasant feelings, at least temporarily. Many group members are not used to managing distress or handling feelings while being drug free, so this is often difficult at first. Negative emotional states and the inability to manage

them effectively account for the largest percent of relapses to substance use following a period of recovery (Daley and Marlatt 1997). Group members often benefit from learning basic emotional management skills such as being able to identify and recognize feelings, accept them, and learn to live with them without escaping to substance use.

8. Boredom with recovery and the feeling that life isn't much better despite being off of drugs: Many cocaine dependent individuals like excitement, action, and "living on the edge." Recovery is a major adjustment for them. It often is much less exciting than the feelings produced by cocaine use, wheeling and dealing on the streets, "getting over" on other people, and partying. Some members also experience boredom with relationships, their job, or other aspects of life.

9. Psychiatric disorders or other types of addictions: Psychiatric disorders are common among clients with cocaine addiction (Weiss and Collins 1992; Beeder and Millman 1997; Sterling et al. 1994). In some instances, group members will have comorbid psychiatric disorders, such as mood or anxiety disorders, that contribute to their difficulty with emotional states, interfere with recovery, cause personal distress, or contribute to suicidal feelings. Some members also have other addictions or excessive behaviours, such as compulsive gambling, sex, spending, or work habits. While the group is not intended as a therapy group for mental health disorders, psychiatric problems may be discussed in the context of recovery from addiction. The group counsellor should encourage members with diagnosed psychiatric disorders to talk about their mental health problems or concerns with a mental health professional. However, if members are not in treatment, the group counsellor should encourage them to get an appropriate evaluation to determine if psychiatric treatment is needed.

10. Other psychosocial problems related to school, work, housing, finances, the legal system, or how to structure leisure time may also be discussed in group sessions.

FAMILY INVOLVEMENT

Cocaine addiction contributes to a variety of family difficulties, affecting the family system as well as individual members. The burden and emotional pain can be great. Family members may exhibit behaviours intended to help the addicted member, but which ultimately have an adverse impact. Family involvement is important in the treatment of addiction (O'Farrell and Fals-Stewart 1999, pp. 287-305).

There is an association between relapse and social supports across a range of addictions. Involving the family or significant other of the addicted client in individual or multiple family group sessions can reduce the risk of relapse. Such involvement has many potential benefits:

— It provides the counselling staff with an opportunity to learn about the client's family, observe how family members interact, and gain input from the family.

— It can facilitate compliance with treatment. If a client feels pressure to remain in treatment to satisfy the requests of the family, he or she may maintain this involvement even during periods of low motivation. This buys the client time for motivation to improve.

— It provides members of the family with an opportunity to verbalize their concerns, questions, experiences, and feelings related to the addicted family member.

— It offers the client an opportunity to hear how the family experiences the addiction.

- It offers the client the opportunity to receive support from the family.
- The family can receive education and support from other families, which may lessen the burden experienced. Anger, worry, confusion, and other emotional reactions can be shared, and strong, negative feelings may be diffused.
- Family members can be taught about and encouraged to attend support groups such as Nar-Anon or Al-Anon.
- Family members can learn about behaviours that they should avoid, which are considered enabling.
- Family members can learn about strategies that can help them cope better with an addicted relative.
- Family members can learn about strategies to take care of themselves so that all the recovery efforts are not simply directed at the addicted person.
- Family members with a psychiatric or addictive disorder who appear to need help themselves can be encouraged to seek help, and referrals can be facilitated.

The GDC model includes a one-time Family Psychoeducational Workshop (FPW) conducted during the first month of treatment (Daley and Raskin 1991; Daley et al. 1992). Psychoeducational workshops have been used with all types of psychiatric and addictive disorders. Such workshops have a positive impact on participants by lessening the family's burden, increasing helpful behaviours, and decreasing unhelpful behaviours.

A variety of formats can be used for FPWs. Although the CCTS offered a single, 21/2 hour FPW workshop, these workshops can be offered for longer periods of time or for more than one day. A brief FPW was necessary in the CCTS because of the research design. Because the CCTS focused on evaluating the efficacy of individual treatments for addiction, an extensive family programme would have made it difficult to interpret research findings. In community-based programmes, however, using a variety of family approaches is recommended, including multiple family groups, family psychoeducational workshops, individual family sessions, sessions with individual family members based on a specific need, and referral to family-related self-help programmes.

Family Workshop Content

The specific material covered in family psychoeducational workshops will depend on the amount of time available. Following are the topics most commonly addressed in the CCTS family workshops:

- Overview of substance abuse and dependence: Prevalence, symptoms, causes, and basic concepts (e.g., various degrees of substance use problems, denial, obsession, compulsion, tolerance, psychiatric comorbidity, etc.).
- Effects of substance use disorders: Impact on the individual, family system, and individual members, including children.
- Overview of recovery: Recovery issues for the affected person (physical, psychological or emotional, social, family, spiritual, other) and how to measure outcome.
- Overview of treatment resources: Treatment approaches for the affected individual and treatment resources.
- How the family can help: Enabling behaviours for the family to avoid, and behaviours that are helpful in supporting the addicted family member's recovery.

— Family recovery issues: How a family member can heal from the adverse effects of addiction and involvement in a close relationship with an addicted family member.
— Self-help programmes: Programmes available for addicted clients and family members, how they can help, and how to gain access to them.
— Relapse: Common warning signs of relapse, the importance of relapse prevention planning, how the family can be involved, and how to deal with an actual lapse or relapse of an addicted family member.

Family Educational Materials

Families benefit from written information on any of the topics listed above. Families can continue to read and learn about addiction and recovery if written materials are provided or recommended. In addition, educational videos provide an excellent mechanism to gain information and insight, and they often facilitate excellent discussions among families.

Format of a Family Psychoeducational Workshop

FPWs are semi-structured sessions in which a group of clients and their families are provided with specific information about addiction and recovery. Support is also provided, and families are encouraged to share their questions, concerns, and feelings. Because this is not a therapy group, the workshop leaders must make sure that it doesn't become a context for sharing deep-seated emotional feelings. Strong feelings are always present in these workshops, and some sharing of emotion is necessary. However, opening up families too much can be counterproductive, so education and support are the main areas of focus. Interactive discussion is encouraged in the context of increasing participants' understanding of addiction and recovery.

Educational videotapes can be used to help present information and stimulate discussion. It is helpful to provide written literature to clients that relates to the workshop content. Usually after a FPW, one or more family members will have personal questions or concerns that they wish to discuss with the workshop leader.

5

Evaluating Behavioural Change Data and Surveys

OPERATIONAL APPROACHES FOR EVALUATING INTERVENTION STRATEGIES

Audience-Centered Communication

Audience-centered communication is an approach to BCC based on a model of dialogue between those who wish to promote behaviour change and a participating audience. It is essentially a consultative partnership, focusing on interaction at every stage between the communicating institution and the public. While a number of methodological tools are available (focus groups, key informant interviews, and various participatory learning and action [PLA] techniques, among others), no technique will be truly effective unless it is imbued with an attitude of respect for the target audience and a determination to understand the audience's point of view and address the audience's central concerns throughout the BCC campaign, culminating in its evaluation.

Audience-centered communication has three stages. The first stage determines the parameters for effective BCC through a series of research and planning activities. During this stage, communicators look at research already done, and, if necessary, carry out two types of formative research: a situation analysis and an audience analysis. The second stage involves developing a communication concept and messages based on the formative research findings, drafting materials, and pretesting them with the target audience. The third stage involves implementing BCC activities, and includes monitoring communication activities, checking comprehension, and assessing communication effects. While evaluation is often considered a separate phase that follows implementation, experience shows that it is more useful to think of it as an integral part of a communication intervention. This emphasizes the need to generate immediate feedback, verify comprehension, and develop an awareness of effects. The steps of the audience-centered communication cycle are listed below. Activities with a particular relevance to evaluation are in bold face.

I. Planning BCC

Review baseline data

Conduct situation analysis

Segment the audience

Designate target audience(s)

Establish behaviour change goal

Conduct audience analysis

Develop BCC objectives

Make action plan

II. Developing BCC

Develop BCC concept

Develop messages

Choose channels

Develop BCC materials

Pretest BCC materials

Produce BCC materials

III. Implementing BCC

Carry out BCC activities

Conduct process evaluation

Assess communication effects

The evaluation activities conducted at each of these stages are described in greater given in this study.

Evaluating Behaviour Change Communication Interventions

This study will look at the essential evaluation activities performed at different stages of implementing behaviour change communication (BCC) projects and discuss critical issues and inherent challenges. Behaviour change communication is one component of behaviour change interventions (BCI), a broader designation that includes many other types of interventions, such as services, commodity distribution, and community mobilization, in addition to communication interventions.

The evaluation of a BCC project is an integral part of its design and must be considered at different stages throughout the project's development: during the stages of formative research (situation analysis and audience analysis), during pretesting, while monitoring implementation, as well as during the evaluation of communication effects. In other words, evaluation of BCC projects must be considered an integral part of the audience-centered communication cycle, with implications for each of these stages.

Planning BCC

Two types of formative research should be conducted at the planning stage of a BCC project to gather information to guide the project strategies. Planners need to investigate both the individual and community environment before formulating a strategy for behaviour change communication. This research is the basis for developing communication objectives–the criteria on which the BCC project ultimately will be evaluated.

Conduct Audience Analysis

The situation analysis describes the community and larger environment within which change takes place, but ultimately much of the behaviour change with respect to HIV/AIDS and STIs takes place on an individual level. Behaviour change is usually not a one-time, definitive event, but rather is preceded by a series of steps, including changes in knowledge, shifts in attitude, and tentative preliminary steps to behaviour change, such as trying a behaviour once. For this reason, developing an effective BCC programme requires an in-depth "insider" understanding of the members of each of the target audience segments and where the segment as a whole is on the steps of change at any specific time–their level of knowledge, their relevant attitudes (beliefs, values, preferences, expectations), the barriers to change they face and express, and the factors that might motivate them toward behaviour change (as well as their communication preferences, essential information for a strategic choice of channels.)

The audience analysis should seek to provide a clear picture of the interior reality of members of each segment and should provide answers to the following questions:

- How do members of the target audience segments conceive of HIV/AIDS and STIs?
- Where are they in the process of behaviour change?
- What is their level of knowledge of the specific facts

of HIV/AIDS and STIs, their transmission and prevention?

— What is their estimation of their personal risk of becoming infected with HIV and STIs? If they feel they are not at risk, why not?

— What are their perceptions of peer and social norms governing sexual behaviours and HIV prevention?

— What peer groups and significant others are most important to them?

— What are the behaviours that put them at risk for HIV and STIs?

— How do they currently understand and practice preventive behaviours?

— What do they see as the benefits of changing their behaviours?

— What do they see as the disadvantages of changing behaviour? What pressures make it difficult for them to change their behaviours?

— What power do they believe they have to change their behaviour, and if it is limited, why, and by whom or what?

— What would it take for them to change to a safer behaviour or continue with safe behaviour?

— When and where do they usually get information about sexual and health topics?

— How do they communicate with others? Where do they meet? When? Who is in their immediate social network?

— What sources of information on sex and health do they find most credible?

— When and where would be the best times to talk

with them about HIV prevention, distribute condoms, make STI treatment services available, and who would do this most effectively?

Conduct Situation Analysis

The situation analysis (also called community investigation) reveals the parameters within which BCC will take place. It includes an analysis of the:

— Demographic environment–The population in terms of size, density, location, age, gender, race, occupation, education, income, family composition, and other statistics.

— Epidemiological environment–The incidence and prevalence of sexually transmitted infections (STIs), including HIV, among various target audiences.

— Economic environment–The factors that affect people's purchasing power and spending patterns, which will permit a better understanding of how, for example, prostitution, condoms, and health care are purchased. An understanding of the macroeconomics of a country helps explain the role that the infrastructure, the media, and the market will play in distributing health care messages and facilitating programmes.

— Political environment–The laws, government policies, agencies, and advocacy groups that influence and limit various organisations and activities. The political environment can affect condom advertising, public health, access to health care, the economic power of women, the sex trade, sex education, the operation of STI clinics, and the illicit drug trade.

— Cultural environment–The institutions and other forces that shape society's basic values, perceptions, preferences, and behaviours. Religion, language, educational institutions, literature, popular music, the press, and theater all play a role in determining the status of women and in influencing sexual behaviour, attitudes toward AIDS, and family values.

— Organisational/development environment–The programmes, projects, and interventions that are already in place so that complementary and/or shared efforts can be encouraged and duplication avoided.

The situation analysis tells how the community is organised and how it works–essential parameters within which any BCC activity must function. A carefully conducted situation analysis can save time and money by helping to ensure that BCC activities are chosen well and that they correspond to the realities of the situation, avoid traps, and make best use of their opportunities. It also takes into consideration the need to create a supportive environment, which may lead to a focus on advocacy or community development issues needed to support the individual changes BCC is promoting.

On the basis of the situation analysis, the BCC planning team can segment the audience, and choose target audiences from among the segments for specific BCC activities. A target audience is defined as the group that needs to change its knowledge, attitudes, or behaviours to achieve the programme goal. Target audiences for effective BCC include not only groups at risk because of their behaviour, but also others who have an impact on the risk situation, including authorities (such as police), gatekeepers (such as brothel owners), and service providers (such as STI clinic staff).

Develop BCC Objectives

On the basis of the situation analysis and in-depth audience analysis, the BCC planning team then develops communication objectives. These objectives should specify the nature of the change the BCC campaign will engender. They should not be limited to behaviour changes but should also include changes in knowledge, attitudes or the decision or intention to try behaviours that precede definitive behaviour change. Experience shows, for example, that it is often unrealistic to expect that a BCC campaign will bring about an immediate increase in condom use, but a lack of change in condom use does not necessarily mean that nothing has changed. Important changes may have occurred and may be preparing the way for later behaviour change. The process of behaviour change is complex and incremental, and BCC planners can best approach it on those terms–like chipping away at a big stone, rather than trying to move it with a single push. Well-formulated BCC objectives recognize these steps of change.

Knowledge changes are the easiest to identify, and as a result, many BCC campaigns focus on increasing knowledge long past the time when lack of knowledge is really the problem for a target audience. Attitude changes are often even more important but neglected by communicators. For example, audience members may change their idea of condoms from a pregnancy prevention device, to something that can keep them safe from STIs and HIV, or they may increase their personal perceived risk of HIV/AIDS. Norms may also change; it may become more usual for women to negotiate the terms of sexual behaviour as the result of a BCC campaign, or people may develop new concepts of masculinity, or a sense that condoms can be sexy. There may also be changes in law or policy, or changes in the public discourse, as reflected in the media.

Communication objectives should be stated in the future tense, in terms of changes in knowledge, attitudes, and skills or in the policy environment that will be evident after the BCC activity, and they should directly reflect needs identified through the in-depth audience analysis. Here, for example, are some communication objectives aiming at changes that precede behaviour change. Note that they are stated in behavioural terms so that their success is easy to measure:

— Change in knowledge–After the mass media campaign, audience members will say they cannot get HIV through haircuts, manicures, or mosquito bites, or by sharing clothes or dishes.

— Change in attitude (beliefs)–After the campaign, when asked what they think of when they hear the word "condom," audience members will more often use words reflecting a positive image of strength and protection.

— Change in attitude (perceived risk)–After the workshop, audience members will say it is quite possible that they or their friends could get HIV if they have sex outside of a monogamous relationship and do not use condoms.

— Change in skills–After seeing the video and practicing with the peer educator, audience members will be able to show how they would negotiate condom use with a partner.

— Change in the discourse–After the campaign, a survey of the popular press will reveal less judgmental language applied to sex workers.

Developing BCC

Pretest Communication Materials

Once the BCC planning team has written communication objectives, developed concepts, chosen the media channel(s), designed messages (that is, the specific words and images) to express the concept, and developed prototype materials to match the objectives, the materials must be pretested with the target audience. Pretesting is an evaluation activity that gives immediate feedback on the effectiveness of BCC messages and materials. It is an early evaluation of the BCC planning process that can and should lead to immediate adjustments in the materials or methods to be used in the BCC project.

Thorough and systematic pretesting is an essential part of marketing and plays no small role in the success of commercial advertising–a success social marketers have emulated. For example, in Nepal's AIDSCAP II project, implemented by FHI, alternative images of a condom were thoroughly pretested to find one that would appeal to a wide spectrum of audience members and would carry a strong association of condoms with AIDS prevention. A number of options were rejected based on the pretests, and the winning image was further refined. The resulting image of "Dhaaley Dai" (Big Brother Condom) shows a smiling, muscular condom character kicking out a small figure representing the virus. It is accompanied by a slogan (rhyming in Nepali): "Wear a condom and drive away AIDS." This message has been widely disseminated in Nepal and has achieved a very high level of recognition. Alternative versions of materials should always be pretested, so that the pretest has meaning. While the pretest may look like an informal discussion, it should be structured around a definite set of questions that reveal the different qualities for which the materials are being tested. For example, interviewers could use the question guide.

Assess Communication Effects

Monitoring an ongoing BCC programme according to the above standards will go far toward developing an understanding of the effectiveness of that programme. However, it is also useful to pause, after the conclusion of a BCC programme or campaign, to take a close look at the net effect of that programme on the target audience. This can be done using quantitative or qualitative methods. It is possible to conduct a systematic, quantitative evaluation of any change in knowledge, attitude, intention, skill, or reported behaviours (actually a measure of norms) if these are defined specifically enough in the objectives, and if an appropriate methodology is chosen (Section III of this book provides more information on the methodologies for measuring behavioural outcomes).

However, this type of outcome evaluation is often not necessary at the individual project level. A simpler method, and one that usually yields richer insights, is to repeat some of the in-depth formative research with different members of the same target audience segments, to identify any evidence of change. This method, called assessment of communication effects, does not attempt to prove that a certain communication campaign caused a certain change (such causality is misplaced, in any case, when dealing with such a profoundly social realm as communication). Rather, it is an attempt to take a second look at the audience, to see how things have changed since the BCC programme began. For example, suppose that a negative image of condoms has been identified as an attitudinal barrier as a result of focus groups or in-depth interviews in which participants referred to condoms in a variety of negative ways, and a campaign has been conducted to change the image of condoms. After the campaign, follow-up focus groups or interviews with the same segments may reveal some change in the discourse on condoms. A striking example from Vietnam came when follow-up focus groups were held after a BCC campaign in which one of the objectives was to give condoms a more friendly, protective, and less medical image. When the groups were asked, "What do you first think of when you think of condoms?" (a question also asked in the original research) many participants responded, "condoms are like a loyal bodyguard." This phrase, echoing a message from the BCC campaign, provided evidence that the campaign had had its intended effect.

Assessing communication effects can also produce data about exposure to media messages, about recall of specific messages, and about the relative impact of different communication channels. An assessment of communication effects not only reflects the success or failure of a previous BCC campaign, but also provides feedback on audience concerns that can be addressed in the next campaign. In this way, the BCC process can become more like a dialogue between the BCC planning team and the audience. Thus, the assessment of communication effects guides future BCC campaigns, closing the planning-implementation-evaluation circle.

This study has shown how evaluation is an integral part of the design of audience-centered communication projects, not only at the final stage but also at other key points during the project cycle. This ongoing concern with evaluation from the outset helps to ensure that the communication activities are structured around a dialogue between the members of the target audience and the BCC planning team. Elements of evaluation are included in the situation analysis and audience analysis (formative research), in setting BCC objectives, in pretesting of materials, as well as in the process evaluation (monitoring of implementation) and the final assessment of communication effects. Assessing communication effects allows the audience to give feedback on the campaign as well as on changes within the audience itself relating to the campaign objectives.

This then allows the BCC team to plan the next campaign. Thus, the final assessment closes the audience-centered communication cycle and assures that the process maintains its essential character of a dialogue between BCC planners and the audience.

Implementing BCC

Conduct Process Evaluation

Process evaluation is conducted throughout the implementation of BCC activities and actively involves key stakeholders, such as project managers, beneficiaries, organisation staff, and donors. This participatory approach to process evaluation allows the stakeholders themselves to identify the essential indicators they want to measure and report on and helps to insure that the evaluation will be relevant and useful for designing future activities. Its purpose is to determine whether activities are proceeding according to the plan and if not, to indicate where changes need to be made. Questions asked during process evaluation obviously reflect the activities of the programme. They might include such questions as the following (for a peer education activity):

- Were peer educators selected, trained, and supervised?
- Are the peer educators performing the duties that were expected of them?
- Is supervision being conducted as planned?
- Are the communication channels being used as planned?
- Have the radio or TV messages been broadcast?
- Was the target audience involved with message development?
- How many target group members have been reached?

Process evaluation can also examine strengths and weaknesses of an ongoing intervention. What follows is an instrument for assessing and monitoring behaviour change communication interventions that sets out standards for effective projects. It then asks specific questions that lead the user to recognize whether the intervention is adhering to the established standards for high-quality BCC interventions. These questions are meant to be asked throughout the implementation of BCC interventions.

Standard 1: Interventions should focus on well-characterized, specific target audiences.

1. Who is the primary target audience for this BCC intervention?
2. Has this primary target group been appropriately divided by segmenting variables? If not, which variables have not been considered that now appear important to the segmentation?
3. Are there other people who influence the primary target group who are not yet being addressed? If yes, who are they?
4. How can the project address these other people?
5. What is the risk behaviour(s) that the primary target audience is practicing? What is the desired behaviour?

Standard 2: HIV/AIDS prevention interventions and messages must be crafted to motivate and appeal to the specific target audience's perceived needs, beliefs, concerns, attitudes, present practices, and readiness to change.

1. What additional knowledge is needed, what attitudes need to change, and which skills need to be mastered before the target audience will be able to adopt the desired behaviour?

2. What are the main messages used in this intervention? Do the main messages address the needed knowledge, attitudes, and skills? If not, what is missing, or what does not match these needs? (To answer this question more specifically, the following additional questions are useful.)
3. What gaps in knowledge appear to influence audience members behaviour with respect to HIV/AIDS/STIs? Do the messages match the audience's gaps in knowledge?
4. What does the audience perceive as its most important needs? Do the messages match the audience's perceived needs?
5. What are the audience's main beliefs related to sexuality and HIV/AIDS/STIs? Do the messages make appropriate use of (appeal or respond to) these beliefs?
6. What are the main concerns of the audience members? Do the messages refer to these concerns?
7. What attitudes presently inhibit change in the audience? Do the messages respond to the attitudes and encourage/model different attitudes?
8. What undesirable behaviours do audience members currently have? Do the messages specifically address the disadvantages of these undesirable behaviours?

Standard 3: At-risk individuals must be provided with both skills and supplies to prevent HIV.

1. Are any new skills needed for the audience members to change? If so, what skills?
2. Do the messages model the needed skills?
3. Are supplies that are needed for safe behaviour available to all the audience members?

4. Are supplies that are needed for safe behaviour affordable for all the audience members?
5. Is STI treatment easily available and affordable for all the audience members?

Standard 4: A supportive environment needs to be created for HIV prevention and for the protection of those infected with HIV.

1. What are the social, cultural, environmental, political, and organisational conditions that may influence the target audience's HIV/AIDS risk behaviours?
2. Does this intervention try to influence these social, cultural, environmental, political and/or organisational factors? For example, does it:
   - support traditional and cultural values that encourage low-risk behaviours?
   - persuade government officials to change public health policies?
   - influence organisation/corporate officials to discontinue discriminatory practices or policies?
   - mobilize support among the general public to work for changes in public policy?
   - promote the social acceptability of alternatives to risk behaviours?
   - protect human rights of all people affected by HIV/AIDS?
   - actively fight discrimination?
   - educate the whole community for care, compassion, and prevention?

Standard 5: Mechanisms need to be created to maintain and sustain HIV prevention behaviours and activities over time.

1. Does this BCC intervention include follow-up mechanisms to reinforce and encourage the maintenance of newly acquired attitudes and behaviours? For example:
   - periodic follow-ups and re-certification of peer educators;
   - HIV prevention messages mainstreamed into school curriculum at all grade levels;
   - campaigns to reinforce messages focused on maintaining new behaviours;
   - annual meetings for organisations working in the HIV prevention area;
   - meetings organised to discuss "lessons learned."

Standard 6: BCC planners should identify and use opportunities to work collaboratively and in different sectors of the community/country.

1. Does this intervention actively collaborate with other partners and implementing agencies?
2. Does this intervention take into consideration activities and materials aimed at this target audience by other organisations?
3. Is this intervention designed to involve the resources and expertise of other individuals and organisations in the public and private sectors?

Standard 7: A monitoring plan is essential to guide the adequate implementation of behaviour change communication projects.

1. Does this intervention have a monitoring budget?
2. Does this intervention have staff available for monitoring and supervision?

3. Have new directions been identified as a result of monitoring? If so, what are they?

METHODOLOGIES FOR MEASURING BEHAVIOURAL TRENDS WHILE EVALUATING PROGRAMMES FOR HIV/AIDS PREVENTION AND CARE IN DEVELOPING COUNTRIES

The Role of Behavioural Research In Monitoring and Evaluation

"Conceptual Approach and Framework for Monitoring and Evaluation," a framework for evaluation was described that included a discussion of the input/output level, as well as that of outcome and impact. The importance of monitoring the resources put into a programme (such as budget and human resources) and the "products" of those inputs (such as availability of condoms and sexually transmitted infection [STI] treatment) were discussed. However, the evaluation of the effectiveness of HIV prevention programmes will almost always require information that informs us about the extent to which the ultimate goals of the programme were achieved. The ultimate goal of most HIV prevention programmes is to reduce the transmission of HIV. So prevention programmes are likely to focus on interventions that will affect the rate of transmission. Among other things, these include encouraging safer sexual behaviour, treating STIs more effectively, and reducing needle sharing between drug injectors. Reductions in the risk behaviours that spread HIV necessarily lead to a reduction in the spread of HIV. For those who are familiar with monitoring family planning programmes, risk behaviours act as the "proximate determinants" for HIV infection. They can therefore act as a proxy for measuring programme impact.

One of the most powerful ways to measure proximate determinants like behaviour change is through repeated quantitative behavioural surveys designed to measure behavioural indicators. The process, also known as behavioural surveillance, is used to track different populations who are exposed to the risk of HIV and whose behaviour may contribute significantly to the spread of HIV. These surveys are conducted to systematically monitor changes in HIV/STI risk behaviours over time, and are conducted at regular intervals (every 1-2 years). There are several reasons for tracking risk behaviours, which vary in importance depending on the type of epidemic in the geographic area of interest, the type of sub-populations that are affected, and the need for data to advocate for an appropriate response. Whether behavioural indicators are measured at the country, district, or project level, they play a role in describing pathways for spread of the virus, guiding programme interventions, evaluating effects of programmes, and increasing the understanding of the epidemic among policymakers and the general public.

Uses of Behavioural Data For Programme Evaluation

Control of the HIV epidemic differs from that of other infectious diseases because of the complex and personal nature of the risk behaviours that drive its spread. An understanding of these behaviours is the key to an appropriate response, and tracking them over time is one of the most crucial elements of an effective monitoring and evaluation system for HIV prevention and care programmes. The purpose of this study is to describe the contribution of behavioural data to monitoring and evaluation, with an emphasis on outcome evaluation. Methodologies that lead to the availability of better quantitative indicators of behaviour change will be discussed in detail. Many different kinds of behavioural research are needed to guide HIV/AIDS programmes in directing prevention resources and helping project implementers plan for appropriate action. Formative behavioural research is needed to help explain the multiple complex factors that influence risk behaviours and to help with the design of effective programmes for specific communities. In addition to helping frame the context for prevention efforts, behavioural research also provides a firm understanding of the patterns and distribution of risk in the population. The systems that are established to monitor these risks feed not only into the design and direction of prevention activities but also into their evaluation.

Seemingly, it would be desirable to have valid and reliable behavioural indicators to evaluate every project that is carried out with a specific sub-population. However, the limited resources for conducting evaluation research and the methodological difficulties involved in gathering high-quality data make this unfeasible in many situations. From the perspective of a national programme, it may not be practical, or even necessary, to assess behaviour change for every individual project, especially when those projects are using strategies with already proven effectiveness. This is especially true in light of the fact that it is usually not possible to attribute to particular interventions changes that have occurred, unless control groups are used. Quite apart from the logistical difficulties of controlled studies, it is usually not ethically feasible to deny an intervention to a control group when that prevention strategy has already been proven effective. Only in the case of a demonstration project to test a new intervention or study an unanswered research question would there be justification for such a rigorous evaluation design.

In situations where there are multiple interventions addressing overlapping sub-populations, it is often more appropriate to combine the resources of comprehensive HIV prevention and care programmes to monitor national or regional trends in behaviours, and to conclude that the changes are attributable to the sum total of programme effort. With regard to individual projects, although there is a need for some behavioural research to help implementing agencies evaluate their efforts in a meaningful way, such research should be consonant with the capacity of the agencies that are carrying out the interventions. It may involve the use of qualitative studies or rapid assessments as opposed to representative, large-scale quantitative surveys.

Informing Effective Programme Design

Effective programme design requires not only a knowledge of who is at risk, but also an understanding of the levels of different risk behaviours. Knowing how much and what kind of risky behaviour people are engaging in helps in setting priorities for intervention needs, and also in gauging how these priorities may change over time. However, knowing levels of risk behaviour alone does not provide the understanding of why people engage in those behaviours and what might motivate them to reduce their risk. Such an understanding is also a critical part of programme design. Each new prevention effort requires careful evaluation of many factors, including social, demographic, and contextual factors. Behavioural research, especially qualitative research, can help provide that understanding, and ultimately help programme managers design interventions that are better targeted to the specific needs of the communities they are addressing.

Explaining Changes in HIV Prevalence Through Data Triangulation

Changes in HIV prevalence may indicate the long-term impact of multiple HIV/AIDS prevention interventions, but it is very difficult to prove that observed decreases in prevalence trends are the result of HIV prevention programmes. Other factors such as mortality, migration, and saturation of the population at risk can also account for such changes. A consensus is emerging among decision-makers that prevention programmes need to investigate both trends in HIV infection and trends in behaviour that may lead to that infection. Indeed, analysed together with other types of information, behavioural indicators can contribute not only to the understanding of trends in the HIV epidemic but also to the understanding of the relationship between programme effort and impact. When behavioural data are analysed in combination with output or process data (such as increased condom availability and improved STI services), and other proximate determinants (for example, decreasing STI rates [other than HIV] and changes in risk behaviours), the evidence that prevention efforts may indeed be having the desired effect is reinforced.

Diagnosing the Problem

One of the most important roles of behavioural surveillance is to provide a "reading" on the levels of risk behaviour existing in communities that are already affected by HIV and to suggest pathways for the spread of the virus. Without some notion of existing levels of HIV and a basic understanding of the potential for spread through high-risk behaviours, public health officials and programme planners would be at a loss to respond, or at least would lack the tools to do so in an efficient manner.

Repeated quantitative surveys can help identify those sub-populations who are most vulnerable to infection, and also indicate the levels of risk behaviour in the general population. Certain sub-populations may interact with people at high risk of HIV infection as well as with people at low risk of infection, thus serving as a behavioural "bridge," potentially carrying the HIV virus from one population to another. Behavioural data collection systems inform public health planners about these networks of risk, helping them to make better decisions about which interventions are most appropriate for various groups, and how to prioritize resources.

Serving as an Evaluation and an Advocacy Tool

A good behavioural data collection system can give a picture of changes in sexual and drug-taking behaviour over time, both in the general population and in vulnerable sub-populations. The system will record a reduction in risky sex just as it will record persistent risk behaviour or shifts in the pattern of risk.

These changes can provide an indication of the success of the overall package of activities aimed at promoting safe behaviour and reducing the spread of HIV. Likewise, they can also indicate areas where current strategies appear to be inadequate or misguided, indicating that alternate approaches or renewed efforts are needed. Showing that behaviour can and does change following efforts to reduce risky sex and drug taking is essential to building support for ongoing prevention activities.

Methodological Issues In Behavioural Surveillance

With this background information in mind, a discussion of current recommendations in measuring quantitative behavioural indicators follows. These recommendations have evolved out of the experience of initiating multiple behavioural surveys in both general population groups and key sub-populations in many different countries.

Planning for Behavioural Data Collection

Consensus Building

Although it has been discussed already in this book, enough cannot be said about the importance of building consensus and gaining support among various partners, including members of the communities involved, local and national health officials, non-governmental organisations (NGOs), and bilateral and international donors/institutions, before proceeding with large (or even small-scale) behavioural data collection exercises. The goals of consensus building are to:

— make clear to the communities who will be the focus of the information gathering how they will benefit from the research and how their cooperation is needed;

— coordinate among government agencies and various donor agencies on plans for large-scale behavioural data collection, seeking input from all the relevant players on decisions about what data are needed, which populations should be studied, and which geographic areas should be covered; this participation will help to use resources efficiently and avoid duplication;

— ensure that the best local researchers are involved and that an appropriate institutional base is established for ongoing behavioural data collection.

Rapid Assessment Through Use of Existing Data

Before planning large-scale data collection, it is particularly important to conduct a rapid assessment of risk behaviours and to map out the location and size of risk groups. Care should be taken to use existing data. Previously existing qualitative research can indicate which sub-populations are most at risk in a society, and can provide a better understanding of these populations that will greatly enhance the planning of the quantitative surveillance activities. More information about rapid assessment and mapping of risk groups.

Choosing Populations to Monitor

Repeated cross-sectional surveys can be conducted in samples randomly drawn from the general population or thought to be representative of the general population. They can also be carried out in selected sub-populations whose behaviour may lead to a disproportionate risk of contracting or passing on HIV infection.

General Population

General population surveys using household-based sampling frames can provide a credible picture of the extent of risk behaviour in the general population and of the links between the general population and groups with higher-risk behaviour, such as sex workers or drug injectors. It is generally recommended that surveys among general population adults take place every 4-5 years. These surveys are important because they provide an understanding of the magnitude of the links between the general population and higher-risk groups that is essential to planning an effective national programme and directing resources. If behavioural data collected in the general population show that links to populations with higher-risk behaviour are limited, then prevention resources can be concentrated largely in more vulnerable populations, with general population efforts being developed more gradually.

Should these links, however, be more extensive, then prevention programmes will need to expand coverage of their efforts more immediately. General population surveys do not necessarily need to be nationally representative in order to be useful to national programmes.

Large, geographically stratified samples in specific regions can provide as much useful information and at a much lower cost. This type of limited survey is recommended unless there are huge behavioural differences between regions, in which case it will be necessary to adjust data collection strategies so that these differences are adequately covered. While it may be easier to conduct behavioural surveys among sub-populations thought to be proxy groups for the general population, such as factory workers, there will always be various sources of bias associated with such populations. Therefore, it is recommended that behavioural surveys in general population groups select respondents randomly from sampling frames composed of households.

Sub-populations with High-risk Behaviour

Household surveys are not adequate for tracking risk behaviours that are not widespread in the general population but which may contribute disproportionately to the spread of HIV, such as injecting drugs, male to male sex, or selling sex. To obtain data from individuals with these high-risk behaviours, special sub-population surveys must be conducted.

Bridge Groups

Household surveys also do not reach individuals who are mobile and who tend to spend extended periods of time away from home, such as the military or migrant workers, long-distance truck drivers, or other frequent travelers. These groups also may be disproportionately likely to contract or pass on HIV, and specific surveys are required to reach them in sufficient numbers.

These groups have the potential to drive the growth of an epidemic, especially in the early stages. If they become infected in large enough numbers, they can act as a conduit of infection between high-risk sub-populations and the general population. Given this situation, it is important to gather information about risk-taking behaviour in these groups, and to design interventions to meet their specific needs.

Youth

Young people are particularly vulnerable, especially in populations where sexual activity begins at an early age. Young people are especially susceptible to HIV in part because they have only recently become sexually active and tend not to be in stable partnerships. It is appropriate to carry out repeated behavioural surveys only in sub-populations that are the target beneficiaries of prevention programmes. Besides being unethical to collect information from a population one has no intention of supporting, it is also pointless.

Firstly, behaviour is unlikely to change substantially in the absence of prevention programmes. Secondly, the purpose of collecting any data is ultimately to inform and/ or improve programming. If no programming is planned, data collection is a waste of time, money, and effort. The choice of which target groups to survey should be driven by the stage of the epidemic. WHO/UNAIDS2 defines the stages of the epidemic as follows:

- Low-level epidemics-Those with an HIV prevalence assumed to be less than 5 percent in all known sub-populations presumed to practice higher-risk behaviours
- Concentrated epidemics-Epidemics with an HIV prevalence that has surpassed 5 percent in one or more sub-populations presumed to practice higher-risk behaviours but that remains below 1 percent among proxy groups for the general population, such as pregnant women.
- Generalized epidemics-Epidemics in which HIV has spread far beyond the
- sub-populations with higher-risk behaviours, which are now heavily infected, and is higher than 1 percent

among proxy groups for the general population, such as pregnant women.

Groups at high risk of contracting or passing on HIV are important to track relatively often at any stage of the epidemic, and bridge groups should be monitored as soon as HIV is detectable in any significant amount among those groups with high-risk behaviour. It is recommended that youth populations be surveyed every 2-3 years once a country has entered into a concentrated epidemic stage in which HIV is present in high-risk groups with whom young people might be interacting. General population household surveys are recommended on a less frequent basis because they are logistically difficult and expensive to carry out. Some of the advantages of non-household surveys are that by going straight to the groups with the higher-risk behaviours, surveys can be done with smaller samples and less movement of survey teams, and therefore can be done more frequently.

However, these advantages are counterbalanced by the fact that high-risk groups outside of households can be harder to reach, in the sense of being more difficult to locate and identify. A great deal of care must be exercised to ensure that systematic and repeatable sampling approaches are used that will help to minimize bias. People often compromise in carrying out behavioural surveys with high-risk groups that are hidden and difficult to identify by using convenience sampling techniques to reach them. The price to be paid for convenience sampling is that one can never be certain about who the data really represent, or whether apparent changes in behaviour are real. Making the effort to be systematic about sampling groups that seem to be disorganised almost always pays major benefits. More details on this subject are included later in this study in the section on "Whom to Survey."

Just as there are groups that are important to survey, it is important to point out that certain groups are inappropriate for behavioural surveillance. Notably, some of the groups that make sense to monitor for HIV surveillance, such as pregnant women and STI clients, make little sense for behavioural surveillance. Asking women in the later stages of pregnancy about their sexual behaviour and condom use will not generally yield results in any way typical of the female population at large. Similarly, if one is trying to measure increases in condom use as a way to monitor reductions in risk behaviour in a given high-risk "source" population, then sampling STI clients to represent the high-risk population produces a built-in selection bias because STI clients by definition are not likely to use condoms consistently.

Considering Measurement Issues

It is important to adhere to a minimum standard of rigor in the conduct of behavioural surveys, if high-quality data are to be obtained. If it is expected that behavioural indicators will shed light on understanding the dynamics and likely future course of localized HIV epidemics, then it must be recognized that it takes time and effort to do good work. Cutting corners and oversimplifying the process in the name of convenience and ease of implementation is ultimately not helpful because the information produced from such research is not meaningful for monitoring behaviour change and evaluating the effects of interventions. In the discussion that follows, three important issues related to collecting high-quality information are discussed. These include:

- what to measure (indicators);
- whom to survey (sampling); and
- how to obtain valid results (validity)

What to Measure

The goal of tracking behaviours in the context of HIV prevention is to learn about behaviours that are critical to the spread of the epidemic. It is very useful to define these behaviours as indicators, so that they may be tracked in a consistent manner over time. Because prevention programmes aim to reduce unsafe sexual and drug-taking practices, indicators are designed to track such key indicators as:

- — reductions in multiple sexual partnerships;
- — increase in condom use with multiple sex partners;
- — delays in the onset of sexual activity (for youth);
- — reduction in sharing of needles (for injecting drug users)

It is worth mentioning that each of these areas represent the very end-stage of behaviour change in most target groups, and that there are many other important knowledge and attitudinal changes that must take place before individuals get to the point of changing these behaviours. Programme planners need to be aware of all the intermediate steps that individuals need to take so that communities can get to these endpoints. Many other behavioural research techniques are available as tools to help assess the needs and progress of communities targeted by interventions. As alluded to earlier in the study, these include formative research using qualitative techniques and rapid quantitative surveys. However, with regard to quantitative indicators, it is important to think carefully about the limited set that are worth measuring, and the hard work required to measure them well. One of the challenges faced in measuring indicators is in knowing how to define such concepts as "high-risk" partners and "condom use." There are many different ways to define each of these. For example, high-risk partners could include paid sex partners or casual partners that one does not know very well. But a supposed "non high-risk partner," such as a spouse, could also turn out to be high-risk, if that person is engaging in unprotected sex with an HIV-infected person. Similarly, there are many different ways to define condom use, including condom use at last sex and "consistent" condom use, which can be thought of as using condoms each and every time there is sexual contact. Condom use is also likely to vary depending on who the sexual partner is, so this must also be factored into the indicator.

Because there are so many different ways to define indicators, it is useful to have a standardized set that can be shared among different groups involved in HIV monitoring and evaluation. Working together to define indicators, it is possible to use collective experience to learn what works well and what does not. Evaluation professionals around the world are pursuing ongoing efforts to refine and improve the recommended set of indicators for monitoring HIV prevention programmes.

The issue of setting targets for indicators. Targets refer both to the magnitude of effect that it is possible to measure and to the level of attainment to be measured by the indicator. The smaller the change it is desired to measure, the larger the sample size that will be needed to do so. This can sometimes pose a problem for evaluators, because it is usually not practical or affordable to work with large samples. This means that if small changes are occurring, such as a 5 percent increase in the percent of men who used a condom the last time they had sexual intercourse with a high-risk partner, or a 5 percent decrease in the proportion of men visiting commercial sex workers in the past 12 months, these changes might not be detectable with the usual sample sizes. Or, if they were detected, they might not be considered significant in a statistical analysis. It is easier to measure larger changes, but prevention programmes may not be capable of achieving those large changes, especially during short periods of time. In these instances, what may look like programme failure may really be a failure of the methodology to be sensitive enough to measure the change. In addition, despite our best efforts, we do not always know how much behaviour change is reasonable to expect in different settings and among different populations because of the complex and unpredictable nature of human sexual behaviour.

We must therefore exercise caution in not over-interpreting behavioural indicators, and also in setting reasonable measurement goals in terms of feasibility and cost. It is generally recommended that repeat surveys attempt to measure change on the order of 10-15 percentage points. However, it is most useful to look at the trends over several rounds of data collection rather than to focus on the difference between any two specific data points. This is because of the strong possibility that any individual data point might well be the result of random fluctuation or chance. It is better to rely on several data points to tell the story than just one or two. This is where the real power of repeated measures comes into play.

It must also be kept in mind that at a given point in time, indicators may reach their maximum levels of change, at which point the focus must switch to the equally important event of sustaining behaviours at their present level. When indicators are close to their optimum value, it becomes futile and impractical to keep trying to measure smaller and smaller increments of change. If, after several rounds of behavioural surveillance, behaviour changes seem to be leveling off, it may be time to reduce frequency from once a year to once every 2 years. If, on the other hand, risky behaviours persist at high levels, then renewed intervention efforts and continued behavioural surveillance are called for.

Whom to Survey

The issue of how to sample "hard-to-reach" target groups, such as injecting drug users, sex workers, and in particular, mobile and migrating populations, is one of the most difficult challenges that exists for those involved in behavioural surveillance. Although it is frequently said that it is not possible to do random sampling with these "moving targets," it is definitely possible to use sound, systematic sampling approaches. Such approaches, if used consistently from one round to the next, increase the likelihood of obtaining reliable estimates of indicators with a minimum of bias. Given the urgent need for scientifically defensible data on behavioural trends in the groups most affected by the epidemic, there is a need to move from non probability-based to probability-based sampling to the extent feasible.

It is not always necessary to have a comprehensive list of all sub-population members to do probability sampling. In fact, because of the sensitive nature of the data being collected, which in many instances involves identifying individuals engaging in illicit behaviours and interviewing them about those behaviours, it is, in fact, preferable not to have a list. This is because of the imperative need to respect the privacy and ensure the confidentiality of all respondents who give their consent to participate in behavioural surveys. All that is needed to do probability sampling is information (or maps) of sites where individuals from the sub-population in question can be accessed. Probability methods can be used for all groups for which a sampling frame of sites or locations where group members congregate can be constructed. For groups for which sampling frames of sites/ locations cannot feasibly be created, network or snowball sampling approaches can still be used in such a way as to improve the reliability of estimates.

How to Obtain Valid Results

Equally as challenging as sampling hard-to-reach groups is the quest for valid results. If it cannot be assured that the data collected are meaningful, then it does not matter how perfect the sampling may be. The results will still not be useful. Apart from sampling error and selection bias, two main sources of error interfere with the ability to gather valid data. One comes from the people collecting the data and the other from the survey respondents. Both contribute to systematic error and both are avoidable if care is taken to exercise quality control during fieldwork.

It is commonly said that people do not tell the truth about their sexual behaviours, and that they exaggerate, withhold information, or refuse to admit to behaviours that are culturally unacceptable. Women, especially, are thought to be reluctant to talk about sex. However, interviewing techniques exist that increase the likelihood of honest sharing of information. Well-trained interviewers who are well-equipped to handle situations that arise in the field are generally able to encourage honest responses and collect data that are credible and consistent with evidence from other sources.

To increase the likelihood of honest responses, interviewers must be thoroughly trained in open and non-judgmental questioning techniques and in accurate recording of responses. The amount of training required will vary depending on who is carrying out the survey. Where peers of those in the respondent group are selected as interviewers, they may be less likely than professional researchers to appear judgmental. Without adequate training they may, on the other hand, also be more prone to recording or coding responses in a way that reflects their own opinions or behaviour. Sometimes, using same-sex interviewers or members of the sub-population, such as MSM or IDUs, to interview other members of those sub-populations can make the total difference between being able to obtain valid information or not. There is some evidence that use of computer-generated questionnaires also improves the likelihood of valid responses9. During the stage of adapting the questionnaire and organising the fieldwork, these aspects of the survey, such as the profile of interviewers for obtaining the most valid results, the proper environment for conducting interviews, and the time it takes to complete the interview should be pretested. At this stage, it is sometimes necessary to conduct some focus group discussions or in-depth interviews with members of the target group to understand ways to improve validity of responses.

Building rapport with sub-populations with whom behavioural research is being conducted is an essential element of success. When researchers have not worked closely with marginalized communities or taken the time to build support for the research process, the result is very often a lack of cooperation and ultimately an inability to obtain high-quality information. There are great benefits to building the support of the communities being studied by involving them in the research process. In addition to getting more meaningful information for monitoring behaviour change and evaluating the effects of prevention efforts, learning to access and build trust in the communities to be surveyed will open the doors for later prevention efforts. Failure to do so can backfire severely and contribute to an atmosphere of hostility and distrust that can last for several years.

Among the numerous issues that can help to obtain valid survey results, many relate to the survey instrument itself. Some things that can be done to improve questionnaires are:

— conducting qualitative research before the survey to learn about some of the characteristics of the target group, and how best to approach them;
— comprehensively adapting and pretesting questionnaires so that they are suited to the local context;
— verifying that the language in the questionnaires is clear to the people being interviewed and that the questions are answerable;
— taking the time to do translation and back-translation to make sure that complex concepts are interpretable in a commonly understood manner; and
— using self-or computer-administered questionnaires when dealing with literate populations.

There is some evidence to suggest that people do respond more truthfully when self-administered questionnaires are used, as opposed to face-to-face interview9. However, it is not always necessary that the whole questionnaire be self-administered. Sometimes it is enough for only the most sensitive questions to be self-administered. The important thing is that that the same method of questioning, whether it be self-administered or face-to-face, be used for each respondent in a given sample population.

Other quality control issues relate to interactions with the groups being surveyed. Often these surveys are conducted among communities that are on the margins of society or the law, and therefore reluctant to open up to strangers. Working through NGOs who have relationships with the populations in question is an essential component of this work. In some cases, such as with MSM or IDUs, it will be necessary to use members of the community itself (or those working with them) to do the interviewing.

In terms of the actual data collection, care must be taken to ensure that interviews are conducted in strict privacy and out of the earshot of friends and family members. Intensive supervision of interviewers by experienced staff is also a necessity.

Despite the best efforts to control the fieldwork, the nature of self-reported data is such that it is not possible to verify the results objectively. Therefore, it is necessary to use more than one method to assess behaviour change-the concept of multiple method triangulation. In the case of behavioural surveillance, it involves the use of qualitative methods after the survey to help interpret the findings. It also involves the use of biological data (HIV and STI prevalence) and other data, such as recorded condom sales or increased use of STI treatment facilities, to validate the findings of behavioural surveys.

Meeting Special Challenges

Although household surveys with general populations have been conducted for a number of years in many countries in the context of evaluating HIV prevention programmes, the experience of repeating surveys among hard-to-reach populations with higher levels of HIV risk is new to most countries. Such surveys require skill, sensitivity, and the backing of the communities involved, all of which take time to develop. Some of the special challenges involved in doing these surveys are discussed below.

Who Should Conduct the Research?

Developing the technical capacity of a local institutional base to conduct behavioural surveillance is of paramount importance to ensure continuity over time. The involvement of independent private research firms without a vested interest in the continued use of the data can be problematic and can threaten the sustainability of the system. While this does not necessarily have to be the case, it is clear that without sufficient capacity building and commitments from the national government and international donors, a high-quality surveillance system cannot be maintained. In addition, although many countries are increasing their focus on decentralisation and participation at the regional, district, or provincial level, including supporting surveillance, a need still exists for a solid institutional base at the central level to maintain national standards. In some countries, this is being handled by making provincial AIDS committees central to the data collection process and by training a team of interviewers at the local level who can be involved in surveillance on a continual basis from one survey round to the next.

Ethical Issues for Hard-to-Reach Groups

Ethical issues are always a concern, but may be even more of an issue when dealing with some of the high-risk groups that are most at risk of HIV. Confidentiality is important for all survey participants, but when the participant of the survey is a group involved in illegal activities, such as sex work, injecting drug use, or illegal migration into another country for work, the importance of protecting privacy is magnified. Sometimes, the factors that make these groups so hard to reach are the very ones that put them at elevated risk of HIV infection in the first place. Yet if they were to be sidestepped for collecting information simply because they are difficult to access and complicated to deal with, then this would be tantamount to sidestepping the epidemic itself.

Researchers must be highly sensitive to the reality

that for some of the groups being studied, the survey itself could pose a danger because it might expose members of the group to authorities who would fine or imprison them. Social discrimination as a side-effect of the survey also cannot be easily controlled. Even if results cannot be linked to individuals, if they are linked to a community of people, they can still be quite damaging, and provide the impetus for increased stigmatisation. Special efforts must be made to ensure that survey participants understand their rights and the risks involved, and that every effort is made to ensure that the community will benefit from the data collection effort. One of the simplest, but often overlooked ways to do this, is to involve the community in planning the survey and in disseminating its findings. This can help reduce the perception, frequently held by target groups, that they are merely being used as sources of information that will ultimately benefit other groups.

Some of the reasons for this are that:

— HIV surveillance and behavioural surveillance have different measurement objectives, usually with different sample sizes and some differing sub-populations;

— refusal rates for biological testing and behavioural surveys can be very different; and

— collecting biological specimens accompanied by detailed behavioural information makes it more difficult to ensure confidentiality

When all is said and done, the logistical and ethical difficulties involved in combining these surveys should be considered in light of the value added, which may be negligible in comparison to the benefits of doing them separately.

It is fair to say that behavioural data provide some of

the most useful information available in the fight against AIDS, especially because at present, behaviour change is the only weapon available for breaking the transmission cycle. However, good behavioural data are not easy to acquire. Without carefully planned data collection strategies and a strong commitment to establishing high-quality data collection systems, programmes will continue to collect volumes of useless data.

Although many different types of behavioural research are needed by HIV/AIDS prevention programmes, collecting high-quality behavioural indicators fulfills many objectives, including monitoring the dynamics of the epidemic, identifying the groups most at risk and helping describe the patterns of their behaviour, and guiding programme planning and evaluating programme effects. One of the most useful and powerful ways to collect behavioural data is through repeated cross-sectional surveys in groups that are important to the spread of the epidemic. Repeated behavioural surveys should be conducted for the general population every 4-5 years and more frequently among high-risk groups that are the focus of HIV prevention efforts. Selecting which target groups to monitor should be carefully thought through, taking into account the stage of the epidemic, the presence of various high risk and vulnerable groups, and the data needs of the country. Because many of the populations that are in the center of HIV spread are difficult to identify and access, attention should be given to working in partnership with the communities at risk, and using systematic, repeatable approaches to sampling and surveying that will produce reliable, valid and unbiased data. Ethical considerations are particularly important because many of the target groups that are most useful to monitor are also highly marginalized groups that are sometimes engaged in illegal activities. Without their trust and cooperation, successful survey work cannot be achieved. Behavioural surveillance is now recognized as an essential component of second generation surveillance that supports the improved interpretation of epidemic trends. Therefore, every effort should be made by countries to establish an institutional base for conducting behavioural surveillance and steps should be taken to strengthen the technical capacity to sustain high-quality data collection systems.

Coordination of Behavioural and Biological Data Collection

It is a good idea to collect behavioural data in the same catchment areas where HIV surveillance is occurring, so that both behavioural and biological trends from the same locations can be observed over time. For the purposes of regular monitoring and evaluation it is not, however, advisable to attempt to collect biological specimens and behavioural data from the same individuals.

INDICATORS AND QUESTIONNAIRES FOR BEHAVIOURAL SURVEYS

This study examines two areas critical to evaluating behaviour change interventions: identifying indicators concerning HIV-related risk behaviour and developing questionnaires to measure those indicators. Since the earliest recognition of the HIV/AIDS epidemic, attempts have been made to identify and define indicators of HIV-related risk behaviour that can be used to measure individual and community levels of risk, as well as to track changes in vulnerability over time. At the onset of the epidemic, a major concern was simply assessing general knowledge and awareness of the epidemic, as well as measuring general patterns of sexual behaviour. Over time, and with the development of comprehensive HIV prevention and AIDS care programmes, the need has been increasingly felt for more detailed indicators that can assess the subtle aspects of behavioural responses to the epidemic as well as help identify obstacles to behaviour change.

As the understanding of the HIV epidemic has deepened and the sophistication and orientation of HIV-related programming has developed, it has become increasingly clear that the epidemic cannot be considered from a static perspective in which all epidemics in all settings are considered to involve the same elements and dynamics. Rather, a more targeted approach has been developed, which considers the epidemic in three stages:

— Low-level–HIV prevalence has never risen above 5 percent in groups of people with known high-risk behaviours, including sex workers, injecting drug users, and men who have sex with men.
— Concentrated–HIV prevalence has risen above 5 percent in at least one of the groups known to have high risk behaviours, but remains below 1 percent among sexually active adults in the "general population" (represented by antenatal clinic clients).
— Generalized–HIV prevalence among sexually active adults in the general population has surpassed 1 percent.

In considering these stages, considerable effort has gone into better defining the critical groups whose behaviours should be tracked over time as well as the indicators used to measure these behaviours. For example, in a concentrated epidemic, priority would be assigned to tracking the behaviours of high-risk sub-populations (such as sex workers and migrant men), whereas in a generalized epidemic, more emphasis would be placed on identifying and tracking risk behaviours in the general population, along with those of high-risk sub-populations. Consequently, the information provided in this study is presented in the context of these developments. In addition, the many lessons learned about how best to ask questions and which indicators provide the most relevant information for measuring change are also presented. Accordingly, this study conveys these lessons and proposes standardized indicators and questionnaires appropriate to the stages of the epidemic as well as to the potential sub-populations most important in the epidemic's dynamic.

These recommended indicators and questionnaires have been refined over time in collaboration with a variety of national and international partners, in a global initiative to determine a minimum set of key indicators for use in evaluating national HIV/AIDS programmes. This key group of indicators is presented here, as well as other indicators deemed important for collecting more detailed data concerning HIV/AIDS-related behaviours.

Developing And Identifying Indicators For HIV/AIDS Behavioural Surveys

Because of the difficulty in measuring HIV incidence directly, as well as the difficulty in using HIV prevalence as a proxy for incidence, behavioural indicators have been heavily relied upon to help predict and monitor the course of the HIV epidemic. Monitoring risk behaviours (such as the frequency of unprotected sex with non-regular partners) over the short and medium term provides a means of assessing changes in behaviour that might influence the course of the epidemic. The adoption and use of a limited set of behavioural indicators that are sensitive to the dynamic aspects of the HIV epidemic over time is therefore critical to the work of programme planners, managers, and evaluators faced with few other interpretable tools. For an indicator to be useful in a national, regional or local programme, it must meet the following criteria:

— An indicator must measure a concept that is relevant to programme effort.

— A programme must be undertaken that proposes to effect change in the concept being measured (there is no point in measuring something that is not expected to change over time).

— The indicator must be able to measure trends over time.

— It must be feasible to collect data for reporting the indicator.

— The indicator must measure only one concept at a time and be easy to interpret.

These indicators are mostly related to sexual behaviour, focusing on number and types of partners and condom use. But in many parts of the world, in addition to sexual transmission, transmission through sharing needles is also responsible for a considerable proportion of new HIV infections.

Therefore, indicators relating to sharing drug injecting equipment are included as well. While it may be desirable to monitor indicators concerning knowledge and attitudes (especially in the areas of stigma and discrimination), including questions related to these areas will be a matter of choice depending upon the focus of a particular programme.

Indicators presented in this study are divided according to sub-population group of interest, including adults ages 15-49, unmarried youth, female sex workers, men who have sex with men, and injecting drug users. All indicators should be measured and reported by gender, as it is widely recognized that risk behaviour characteristics tend to vary greatly between men and women.

Key Indicators In Assessing Behavioural Risk

Indicators most relevant to programming for HIV/AIDS and sexually transmitted infections (STIs) are those related to sexual behaviour, partner networking, and drug injecting. Information on partner types and multi-partner behaviour (including multiple regular partners, non-regular partners, and commercial partners), the frequency of sex, partners' sexual behaviours, and the timing of multiple partnerships (concurrent or serial) are important factors to consider when attempting to understand the level of risk and vulnerability of different groups. Unfortunately, however, the choice of key indicators measuring sexual behaviour can be very complex. The ideal scenario, in which information on every sexual partner and every sexual act over an extended period of time is available, is unrealistic both in terms of the capacity of human memory and the logistical limitations of quantitative surveys.

Thus, the indicators related to sexual behaviour and networking presented here represent a compromise between the ideal and the practical. Indicators related to the percentage of the sub-population who are sexually active, who have more than one partner, who have one or more non-regular partners, and who have engaged in commercial sex, provide information important to understanding sexual norms and practices within a community. The recall period for these indicators reflects practical considerations as well, defining a period long enough to allow for potential change and short enough to allow for reasonably accurate recall. This recall period varies, depending on the sub-population.

Condom Use

Following basic information on sexual partnering and networking, information on condom use is critical to appropriate STI/HIV/AIDS programming. Aside from abstinence, consistent condom use represents the only certain means of preventing the sexual transmission of HIV. Thus, tracking indicators of condom availability and use represents an important means of assessing levels of risk among individuals and communities. Questions concerning condom use can be posed in terms of ever use, frequency of use over varied recall periods (week, month, 6 months, year) or frequency of use during most recent sex act with particular partner types. Each of these methods of examining condom use has strengths and weaknesses. First, while the question of ever use of condoms is very specific, it may not relate to recent changes in HIV-related behaviour, and a one-time ever user of condoms is not guaranteed any assurance of reduced risk of HIV infection. In addition, the use of this indicator is becoming increasingly arcane, as availability of and familiarity with condoms increases globally. Nonetheless, it can be used as a gross measure of population behaviour related to the introduction of condoms in a community where they were previously unavailable. In addition, increases in ever use of condoms without increases in their regular use may point to specific barriers to or dissatisfaction with their use.

Indicators measuring frequency of condom use over a given time period with different types of partners provide additional information regarding risk behaviour. For example, identifying the percent of populations inconsistently or never using condoms can highlight vulnerable populations that may require targeted interventions. Distinct problems are associated with the use of this type of indicator, however. First, categorizing condom use according to frequency is imprecise, and absolute categories such as every time (100 percent of the time) and never (0 percent of the time) may have fewer responses than such categories as almost all the time or sometimes. In an effort to provide adequate (sensitive) response categories for the reporting of condom use, four response categories are therefore suggested: every time, almost every time, sometimes, and never. The use of four categories helps to achieve an improved distribution of responses across categories.

When interpreting condom use data, it is important to also consider partner type and frequency of sex, in addition to frequency of condom use. For example, men with many non-regular partners who report inconsistent condom use are likely to be at greater risk of infection and transmission than men with only one non-regular partner who report inconsistent condom use. At the same time, however, evidence suggests that individuals either adopt consistent condom use or do not, and therefore, knowing the proportion of individuals who have adopted consistent condom use is an important measure for assessing the impact of prevention programmes on communities and predicting future trends in the epidemic, regardless of partner change and sex act frequency.

Measuring the frequency of condom use during the most recent sex act is often used as an internal validity check to the reported frequency of condom use over a long time period. While consistent condom use may be the ultimate goal, measuring condom use for a randomly selected sexual act (most recent) may provide an indication of the general frequency of condom use across all sex acts, and be a more sensitive measure of intermediate change.

When measuring condom use, however, it is essential to measure condom use related to specific categories of partners. Research has shown that condom use varies with the perception of partner, and asking about frequency of condom use over a given time period without specifying the type of partner will increase reporting of inconsistent use.

For example, a person who consistently uses condoms with commercial partners but never uses them with regular partners will report sometimes use, although the risk of unprotected sex with these different types of partners varies greatly. Also, if some individuals are responding to last time use with a regular partner while others are responding to last time use with a non-regular partner, the understanding of the level of risk involved is obscured.

Onset of Sexual Intercourse

Another key behavioural indicator, median age at first sexual intercourse, is often chosen to reflect changes in broad social norms. When considering use of this indicator, it is important to specify the appropriate denominator. For the indicator to accurately reflect changes in the age at first sex among a population, all members of the population must be considered. Thus, the denominator must include those who have not yet initiated sexual intercourse as well as those who have. If only sexually active persons are included in the denominator, and a significant percentage of a specific age group (for example, girls aged 15-19) have not yet initiated sexual activity, the indicator will report a skewed figure of the median age at first intercourse among those sexually active. This figure will necessarily be a lower figure than the eventual median for the age group once all members have initiated sexual intercourse. This problem can be avoided by including all members of the population in question in the denominator.

Injecting Equipment Sharing Behaviours

In epidemics where there is a concentration of HIV infection among injecting drug users, it is important to include indicators that can measure awareness of the risk of unsafe injecting, as well as the frequency of unsafe injecting behaviours. Reduced sharing of injecting equipment and access to sterile injecting equipment are important IDU indicators. Sharing injecting equipment is both the biggest factor for HIV transmission among drug injectors and the most common focus of interventions, especially in non-industrialized countries where there is not a long history of prevention interventions among drug injectors. Measuring levels of sharing will not only serve to alert programme planners about the need for interventions, but can also be used to advocate with policymakers about the need for harm reduction programmes. Changes in sharing behaviour will be especially valuable for tracking trends over time for programmes that support needle exchange initiatives, or that work to improve easy access to safe injecting equipment. When measuring sharing indicators, it is very important to operationalize what is meant by "sharing," because sharing can either be active (loaning injecting equipment) or receptive (borrowing injecting equipment). Being injected by a professional injector or a dealer should also be considered as sharing. Just as with condom use, sharing can be measured either at last injection, or in terms of frequency over time. Because injectors who are addicted tend to inject daily, the time frame for sharing indicators needs to be relatively short–no more than 1 month. Beyond that time period, recall bias becomes an obstacle to valid data. Equally important for IDU populations are those indicators that measure sexual risk-taking behaviours, because sexual partners of IDU are at increased risk of being infected. Also, drug-taking itself may lead to increased likelihood of high-risk sexual behaviour. Reducing sexual transmission should be a primary objective of IDU interventions.

Knowledge

Knowledge indicators have frequently been included in HIV/AIDS-related surveys, but while these indicators are generally useful in measuring overall awareness of HIV/

AIDS information in a community, they often provide only a weak indication of risk levels within a community. An established gap exists between correct knowledge of prevention methods and the use of these prevention methods. For example, even though people know that condoms can prevent the transmission of HIV, it does not mean they correctly or consistently use condoms.

In addition, increasing levels of knowledge over time often means that knowledge indicators are not useful in interpreting risk-related change. For example, early on in the epidemic, the proportion of respondents reporting having ever heard of AIDS was often measured. Now, however, awareness is increasingly widespread and subsequently little change in this indicator can be expected over time in most populations. As a result, knowledge of the existence of AIDS is less and less frequently measured, and has been replaced in many settings by the measurement of accurate knowledge of means of transmission and prevention and attitudes concerning stigma and discrimination. These indicators have been proven to better indicate levels of risk and acceptance of people living with AIDS within a community and, thus, more useful to programme evaluation and planning in the current global context of HIV/AIDS.

Another knowledge area that is often assessed is knowledge of STI symptoms because of the established link between STIs and the increased potential of HIV infection and transmission. The higher the prevalence of unrecognized and/or untreated STIs, the higher the risk of increased transmission and infection due to the presence of STIs. For a population to seek appropriate and timely care for STIs, they must first be able to recognize that they are infected. The behavioural indicator that correlates with this knowledge area is seeking appropriate and timely treatment for STIs. While measuring this indicator is desirable, it is also problematic because the number of respondents reporting having had STI symptoms and having sought treatment is often insufficient to accurately report findings or follow trends over time.

Risk Perception

While programme planners frequently wish to assess risk perception, undertaking this estimate accurately is extremely difficult. First, risk perception must be examined in the context of behaviour in order to be meaningful–without an accurate idea of past and current behaviour, self-perceived risk is difficult to interpret, if not meaningless. But even when assessed in the context of self-reported risk behaviours, "correct" risk perception is difficult to ascertain. For example, a survey among sex workers in Jamaica found that an equal proportion felt they were at risk and not at risk. Subsequent questions determined that of the women who reported nearly 100 percent rates of condom use, half reported that they were at high risk and therefore used condoms, while the other half reported that they were not at risk because they used condoms. In addition, risk perception depends a lot on the stage of the epidemic. In low-prevalence settings, even people with high-risk behaviour may justifiably perceive that their risk is low, whereas in high-prevalence settings, people may already know they are infected (making risk perception for becoming infected irrelevant). In high-prevalence settings, despite having adopted safe sex practices at present, people may perceive that they are at high risk of being infected because of their past behaviours. Finally, it is unclear whether the desirable outcome for this indicator is that it should be increasing or decreasing. It may increase initially, as people become more aware of the risk of HIV infection, but then may decrease again as people adopt safe-sex behaviours. Because of all these ambiguities, assessing risk perception is a complex issue that is more appropriately explored through qualitative research, including focus group discussions and in-depth interviews.

Additional Indicators

A range of contextual factors, such as discussions between regular partners about HIV/STIs, knowledge of someone infected with HIV or who has died of AIDS, regular use of alcohol or drugs, or having been tested for HIV infection, are understood to have a correlation to risk behaviour change. These indicators may be included as additional indicators to allow for a multifaceted examination of determinants of and obstacles to behaviour change. These factors, which relate to the context within which risk behaviour decisions are made, contribute to the improved understanding of the sometimes unclear relationships between knowledge levels and change in risk behaviour. Other indicators that can contribute to the understanding of HIV spread are frequent travel away from home for extended periods of time and age difference between sexual partners. These are not necessarily indicators that one expects to see a change in over time. They merely play a diagnostic role in helping explain the dynamics of the epidemic. Yet another category of indicators are those known as "overlap" indicators. An example of such an indicator would be injecting drug use among sex workers. This type of indicator is meant to raise awareness about the synergistic effects of multiple risk behaviours, and the potential for increased spread of the virus between the IDU network and commercial sex networks. In a similar fashion, it would also be important to measure the extent of sexual risk and selling of sex by a population of injectors.

The indicators recommended here, both the primary and additional ones, are limited in their ability to act as stand-alone measures of the course of the epidemic. However, in conjunction with one another, they provide a comprehensive framework that is useful for analysing risk within a community and comparing risk levels between communities. In the past, quantitative surveys have often been limited in generalizability and replicability because of non-standardized instruments and indicators that restrict comparisons with other data sets. In an effort to diminish the problems associated with variations among and across questionnaires, it is strongly recommended that indicators be selected and constructed in a standardized manner so that an understanding of broad trends in the epidemic can be defined and compared to other populations within the same country, across different countries, and across time.

Determining the Time Frame Of Indicators

One of the most potentially confusing aspects of indicator development is the time frame of behaviours. For example, when asking a male respondent about whether he has had sex with a sex worker, should the time frame for this behaviour be the past month, the past 6 months, or the past year? People tend to remember recent behaviours more accurately and this seems to argue for the use of shorter time frames.

However, if the behaviour is not extremely frequent or common, too short a time frame will yield few respondents and make it difficult to track trends in the behaviour over time with any degree of statistical confidence. Likewise, populations with very frequent risk behaviours will not remember the details of their behaviours over a long time period, such as 12 months. The standardized set of indicators have taken these factors into account, and that is why some are over a 12-month period, while others only consider the past 6 months or the past 1 month. Consistency is critical, because changing the time frame for a behavioural indicator across survey rounds, or deviating from the standardized time frame for a given sub-population will yield dramatically differing results. While different time frames may be appropriate because of differences in local context, it should be kept in mind that comparisons of findings to other sub-populations and settings will be difficult if not impossible. Thus, time frames must be adopted that are both convenient to the respondent and analysable to the researcher.

Developing Questionnaires For HIV/AIDS Behavioural Surveys

Standardized questionnaires should be used for behavioural surveillance to maximise the comparability of data between survey rounds and across sub-populations and geographic regions. Small variations in wording and the order of questions can greatly affect responses to questions so that observed changes in behaviours over time may, in fact, be due to these changes as opposed to any real changes in behaviour. Preparing a well-developed questionnaire that can be maintained over multiple survey rounds with minimal changes is critical, therefore.

International experience in surveying key sub-population groups has generated a wealth of knowledge on what types of questions work and do not work when asking people about their sexual and drug-using behaviours. These questions have been brought together to form questionnaires that, in turn, are used to measure the indicators discussed in the preceding section. These standardized questionnaires have been extensively tested in international settings and are available at Family Health International's website (www.fhi.org) as well as in published behavioural surveillance system (BSS) guidelines. The website also provides information about how and when to use these questionnaires.

Five key sub-population groups are covered by these questionnaires:

— adults 15-49 years old;

— unmarried youth;

— female sex workers;

— men who have sex with men; and

— injecting drug users.

Using standardized questionnaires has many advantages. First, questionnaire development is a difficult process, and already developed instruments such as those cited above contain formulations of questions, time references, and skip patterns that have been tested and are known to produce high-quality data. Second, because these instruments have been used in numerous settings throughout the world, their continued use will allow behavioural surveillance results to be compared internationally to determine differences in the dynamics of behaviour change and the characteristics of different population groups. It is still essential, however, to pretest and adapt survey instruments for every local setting. This involves translating the instruments into local languages and using appropriate local terminology to ensure that the original meaning of the question is not lost. It is also necessary to conduct qualitative research and involve local members of the sub-population groups who can help interpret and adapt the questions and response categories. Back-translating the questionnaire to ensure that the translation into the local language maintains the original version's key concepts and meanings is an important additional step in ensuring the quality of the instrument.

It is also useful to develop a guide for interviewers and supervisors, which goes through the questionnaire one question at a time, explaining in full the rationale behind a question and its intended meaning. This guide can be used in training and in the field, to clarify any ambiguities or misunderstandings that may arise. An example of a supervisor/interviewer guide can be found at www.fhi.org as well as in BSS guidelines.

Informed Consent and Ethical Considerations

Confidentiality and informed consent are important for all research subjects, but when the research involves an illegal or stigmatized activity such as sex work, injecting drug use, or illegal migration, the importance of the privacy of the respondent is magnified.

Thus, behavioural surveys cannot take place without the informed consent of the respondent. Special efforts must be made to ensure that potential respondents understand any risks involved in taking part in the study, and every effort must be made to ensure that the community will derive some benefit from participating in the study. Involving the community in the planning and implementation of the study is one way to achieve this, as is the training of interviewers to ensure that respondents are informed of the purpose of the study and that their participation is requested in a factual and neutral manner.

Measures taken to ensure the confidentiality of the respondent should be explained, and consent should be clearly given by the respondent before interviewing begins. In addition, the interviewer should sign the questionnaire at the time of consent in order to indicate that consent has been given. No respondent names or other identifying information should be recorded. It should be explained to respondents that they have the right to refuse to take part in the study as well as to drop out of the study at any time, and should by thanked politely for their time, whether or not they choose to participate.

Assuring Quality Control Before and During Fieldwork

If care is taken to exercise quality control during fieldwork, two main sources of error that interfere with the ability to collect valid data will be avoided. One source comes from the people collecting data, and the other from the people from whom the data are being collected. It is commonly said that people do not tell the truth about their sexual behaviours, and that they exaggerate, withhold information, or refuse to admit to behaviours that are culturally unacceptable. Experience has shown that certain techniques can increase the likelihood of honest sharing of information. When interviewers are well trained to discuss sensitive behaviours with respondents and make them feel at ease, research suggests that respondents will provide truthful information. Comprehensive interviewer guidelines (such as those cited above) can contribute to the comfort levels of both interviewers and respondents when discussing sensitive topics such as sex and drug taking.

Other quality control issues relate to interactions with the groups being surveyed. Often these surveys are conducted with communities who are vulnerable and therefore reticent to open up to strangers. Working through community organisations that have relationships with the sub-populations of interest in an essential component of ensuring access to community members. In some cases, such as with men who have sex with men and injecting drug users, it is necessary to use members of the community itself (or those working with them) to do the interviewing because it cannot be expected that sufficient rapport can be built between interviewers and respondents in a short period of time. If interviewers do not come from the community, then they must be carefully chosen individuals who will not threaten respondents in any way. Concern for the privacy and confidentiality of respondents and the community must be maintained at all times and winning the trust of the community is essential to obtaining valid results. In summary, key considerations when identifying indicators and developing questionnaires include the following:

— Indicators most relevant to STI/HIV/AIDS programming are those related to sexual behaviour, partner networking, and drug injecting. However, it has become increasingly clear that HIV cannot be considered from a static perspective in which all epidemics in all settings are considered to involve the same elements and dynamics. Therefore it is crucial to consider the stage and location of the epidemic when deciding which indicators to measure.

— When selecting indicators, consider how much a given indicator can be expected to change over time. Some knowledge indicators (or even behavioural indicators) may peak after several years and no longer indicate changes. How the information gathered through this indicator will be used in the programme setting should also be considered.

— Use standardized questionnaires to increase generalizability and replicability across populations and geographic regions and pretest all questionnaires adequately and appropriately.

— Assurances of confidentiality to the respondent and community should be provided.

— All indicators should be measured and reported by gender, as it is widely recognized that risk behaviour characteristics tend to vary greatly between men and women.

— Tracking indicators of condom availability and use represents an important means of assessing levels of risk among individuals and communities. When measuring condom use, it is essential that it be related to specific categories of partners, because research has shown that condom use varies with the perception of partner.

— In epidemics where there is a concentration of HIV infection among injecting drug users, it is important to include indicators that can measure awareness of the risk of unsafe injecting, as well as the frequency of unsafe injecting behaviours.

— Equally important for IDU populations are those indicators that measure sexual risk-taking behaviours, because drug-taking may be associated with increased sexual risk, and because sexual partners of IDU are at increased risk of being infected.

— Regarding timeframes for indicators, people tend to remember recent behaviours more accurately and this seems to argue for the use of shorter time frames. However, if the behaviour is not extremely frequent or common, too short a time frame will yield few respondents and make it difficult to track trends in the behaviour over time with any degree of statistical confidence. Likewise, populations with very frequent risk behaviours will not remember the details of their behaviours over a long time period, such as 12 months. Thus time frames must be adopted that are both convenient to the respondent and analysable to the researcher.

Questionnaire Administration and Interview Settings

In situations in which some members of the sub-population group of interest may be illiterate, data should be collected by a trained interviewer who explains questions to the respondent and records answers. It is important to use the same data collection approach with all respondents because varying the way in which data are collected could bias results (for example, if some respondents are literate and others illiterate, an interview should be conducted with all respondents, rather than self-administered questionnaires being given to literate respondents and interviews conducted with the others). Where respondents are literate and educated (such as in student populations), respondents may record answers to questions themselves on an anonymous written questionnaire, submitting it to a data collection manager in a sealed envelope so that it cannot be distinguished from that of other respondents. It is important to ensure that the style and wording of this type of questionnaire is appropriate to self-administration, and that these questionnaires are pre-tested to ensure clarity and answerability. When using trained interviewers to conduct a survey, it is important for them to conduct survey interviews in a setting where questions and answers cannot be overheard by others as well as to engage in a rapport-building conversation before asking survey questions. This will reduce the likelihood that respondents will give "socially desirable" answers rather than telling the truth. If a third person enters the room or is within hearing distance, the interviewer should explain that it is important to interview the respondent in privacy.

ASSESSING THE VALIDITY AND RELIABILITY OF SELF-REPORTED BEHAVIOURAL DATA

The onset of the HIV epidemic has made the validity and reliability of measurements of sexual behaviours, particularly behavioural change and condom use, critical and salient. The availability of sexual behavioural data is vital to developing and monitoring appropriate prevention programmes, but their effectiveness depends to a large extent on their quality. However, validating sexual behaviour data–in other words, assessing the degree to which reported behaviour reflects actual behaviour–is not easy. The most obvious difficulty is that direct observation or public records are virtually impossible in the context of private sexual behaviour. By implication, sexual behaviour data obtained only through questions represents reported, not observed behaviour. Hence, there is a need for caution in using these data for policy purposes or as the basis of education programmes. For decades, questions on sexual activity have been avoided in most health or fertility surveys on the grounds that such questions were morally and culturally sensitive and the responses were of low reliability and validity. However, many of the problems raised about validity are not specific to sexual behaviours. Questions about child death, fertility, marital status, and income are also highly sensitive.

The extent to which individuals are willing to recall and report details of past sexual behaviour may indeed greatly vary according to gender, age, social status, risk behaviour and many other cultural conditions. In some communities, certain behaviours may be actively concealed because they are illegal or considered socially unacceptable, such as prostitution, homo- or bisexuality, adultery, and premarital sex. In some cultures, men may overestimate their number of sexual partners, and in most societies, women are more likely than men to underestimate their sexual activity outside marriage.

Validity is improved when the research variables to be incorporated in the questionnaire or in the interview guide are tested during in-depth interviews in which the meaning of the language used and the accuracy of recall are checked. Accuracy of recall is an important issue because it can be influenced in a number of ways and it has been shown to vary greatly according to the emotional significance of the event. For example, a person is more likely to accurately recall an emotionally important event, such as age at first sex, than to recall details of regular visits to sex workers. Memory error is more likely to occur for frequent events than for single ones. Respondents with multiple partners may better remember their number if asked to give detailed characteristics of each partner, starting with the most recent one. The reference period should also have meaning for respondents, such as a month, a year or lifetime, rather than artificial periods, such as 3 or 6 months. In addition, a very short reference period may maximise the accuracy of responses but may not capture infrequent behaviours in a particular population.

Pilot testing of the questionnaire should also facilitate decisions about its sequence and structure. It has been shown that validity is improved when the questionnaire is structured in such a way that sensitive questions are asked only to appropriate respondents by using filters and skips, and are placed near the end of the interview. Another issue of sexual behaviour measurement error is the social desirability bias, sometimes called self-presentation bias, that can partly be addressed by careful wording of the questions, by a non-judgmental attitude of the interviewer, and by ensuring maximum privacy.

However, it is also recognized that the social pressure to give desired responses may vary greatly according to the perception of the appropriate preventive behaviours. "Increased" condom use after intense prevention programmes is one example. Several cross-national standard questionnaires on sexual behaviour have been developed in the past 10 years and used in various cultures that have different sensitivities to sexual activity. Core questions about first sex, number of sexual partners, and condom use yield answers that seem to be quite comparable across and within cultures. Other topics, such as commercial sexual contact and risk perception, seem much more ambiguous.

Methods For Checking Validity and Reliability

Several methodologies can be implemented at a minimal cost and contribute to establishing validity and reliability.

Improving Participation Rates

Drawing a probability sample of potential respondents–household- or non-household-based–for surveys of sexual behaviour was long considered an impossible task. However, recent experience has demonstrated that it is feasible and that participation rates in sexual behaviour surveys are as high as in other surveys when several precautions are taken. These precautions also serve to increase the legitimacy of the survey. They are:

- informing the community and the selected individuals or households in advance with letters, radio messages, or community leader visits, and explaining the purpose of the survey;
- selecting interviewers in terms of age, marital status, and gender in order to better match cultural norms on sexual communication;
- training interviewers before going to the field with emphasis on rapport building, talking about sexuality, and overcoming embarrassment;
- including a provision in the survey for a large number of call-backs;
- guaranteeing anonymity and confidentiality to the respondent; and
- ensuring privacy during the interview.

In many developing countries where survey teams have used careful procedures, response rates close to 80-90 percent have been achieved. These rates have been less in urban areas than in rural areas and less in high income areas than in lower. Certainly, although these high response rates are reassuring, they do not guarantee validity if participation is highly selective in terms of risk behaviours.

Consistency with Independent Sources

One of the objectives of most sexual behavioural surveys is to interview a representative sample of men and women. A comparison of estimates of socio-demographic characteristics derived from these surveys (for example, age/sex composition, marital status, urban/rural residence, educational level, occupation) with similar estimates obtained from independent sources of information may provide insights into their representativeness and the extent to which these findings can be extrapolated.

Observed deviations may be due to measurement error and/or sample bias. Non-response rates, including refusal rates and participation bias, are a major concern because of the stigma attached to AIDS. This non-response may simply vary according to repeated absence of families or individuals. In some instances, absence means that selected respondents refuse to participate in the survey. There is limited documented evidence that individuals with high-risk behaviours may be less likely to participate in surveys that address sexual health. However, if HIV/AIDS is explicitly the focus of the questioning, fear and denial may lead individuals with high-risk behaviours to participate less.

Usually, non-response rates are not different for sexual behaviour surveys than for those of other types of surveys using similar methods of sampling. However, because non-respondents in developing countries are often urban male youth and mobile people, their lack of participation may affect the validity of survey results that focus on risk behaviours. Non-household-based surveys, such as school- or workplace-based surveys, that target specific sub-population groups may lead to increased participation if privacy and confidentiality are guaranteed, although the effects of place of interview on validity is still unknown. When comparing socio-demographic indicators such age/sex composition, marital status, urban/rural residence, or educational level with other data sets, other demographic indicators, such as mean or median age at first marriage, may be useful to consider. Median age at first sex and median coital frequency may be added if other data sources exist and if definitions of marriage and first sex are the same in both surveys. The same principles may, in theory, be applied to assess the aggregate validity of sexual behaviour parameters, such as sexual contacts before or outside marriage, reported symptoms of sexually transmitted infections (STIs), or condom use within different partnerships.

However, the possibilities of comparison are usually quite limited because of the absence of independent sources or because of differences in timing of the survey or sampling methods. In a few instances, some data are available in family planning clinics, STI clinics, or health centers, but individuals included in household surveys are likely to be very different from those who report to clinics. Data on condom sales and distribution may be of use, at least as a plausibility check. Commercial sex workers' reports on condom use may be compared with those of clients.

Convergent Validity Checks

Convergent validity is usually used to describe the level of agreement between results provided from different methods of data collection (triangulation), such as face-to-face standard questionnaires, diaries, in-depth interviews, self-completion of questionnaires, or self-completion of sensitive questions (limited to literate populations). Ideally, the comparison should be performed by repeat measures on the same sub-sample and in a short period of time.

However, in the context of sexual behaviour, interpreting differences between different methods is not straightforward because of uncertainty about their relative validity. A high level of consistency between two approaches is reassuring; conversely, inconsistencies should stimulate further research on specific variables. The pattern of inconsistencies might also suggest which method yields more valid information9.

If differences in results are found between structured face-to-face questionnaires and in-depth interviews on the same variables among the same sample population, they may be explained by a variety of factors: the quality and training of interviewers; the time spent to establish rapport and trust-building between interviewer and respondent; the time spent for recall and reflection; the explanation of the meaning of the questions; the flexibility and adaptability of the questioning.

Comparison of daily diaries with retrospective reporting from interviews may provide a useful way of checking recall accuracy. However, willingness to keep sexual diaries might introduce a problem of selection bias10. Qualitative methods usually require the "play-back" method, which means the continual interchange of ideas between investigators and informants and the verification of research hypotheses.

Internal Consistency Checks

A number of internal consistency checks may elucidate the variation of the quality of response over the recall period. These checks depend directly on the type of question asked in particular questionnaires. According to the WHO/ GPA's definition of core prevention indicators, the key variables to assess should include: age at first sex; sex with a non-regular partner in the last 12 months; condom use in the last sexual intercourse with a non-regular partner; reported symptoms of STIs; and knowledge of ways to prevent HIV transmission. Comparisons may thus include: direct versus indirect measure of these specific variables; aggregate reporting of women versus men; aggregate reporting of wives versus husbands (when possibilities exist of linking husband and wife responses). A limited number of aggregate male/female comparisons of coital frequencies and condom use have been made with data sets from five countries where the WHO/GPA protocol was used8. Generally, the correspondence was reasonably high, particularly over short time periods.

Tests of plausibility should also be conducted when associations between variables are known or when different questions on the same topic are asked. For instance, coital frequency between partners usually decreases with the duration of marriage/partnership; age at first sex after age at first marriage should be uncommon; ever use of condoms versus use of condoms as a contraceptive method versus use of condoms as behavioural change due to AIDS may be compared.

Biomedical Validation

Validating self-reports with biological or clinical markers of STIs is a research strategy that has been used in some studies4. Community surveys with appropriate probability sampling procedure and serious ethical precautions may include sampling of blood, urine, or saliva specimens for HIV and STI testing or clinical examination. Such surveys have achieved high rates of participation. Anonymity of the respondent is guaranteed but special procedures may allow researchers to link individual reporting on risk behaviour to biological markers at the data processing stage. However, the major limitation is that the association between sexual partnerships, number of sexual partners, and STIs is far from straightforward. Only a limited number of validity checks may be made using this method, such as consistent condom use versus recent STIs or no sexual activity and the presence of STIs, and even these may be confounded by other factors. Small- or large-scale surveys have an important role to play in monitoring behavioural change over time or to evaluate programme impact. However, despite a growing body of knowledge accumulated on how to conduct such surveys, validity measures are still to a great extent lacking. Obviously, data quality from sexual behaviour surveys critically depends on high standards of execution at each phase of the survey: planning, implementation, analysis, and interpretation. The issue of representativeness of the study population should also be a major concern. Whether the study sample is randomly selected or of convenience, a key factor is to ensure that all reasonable efforts are made to achieve the highest level of response or representativeness, and that the effects of selection bias are documented and integrated into the analysis. This will be critically important to keep consistency between successive surveys.

Indeed, the same type of instrument, interviewer, training, fieldwork strategy, and supervision should be used in successive surveys. This requires a detailed documentation of the baseline survey, including definition of the population of interest and biases in participation. In AIDS surveys, some of the individual characteristics of most concern to the analysis tend to be those associated with unconventional lifestyles and, thus, respondents may be more difficult to reach for interview. This bias cannot be prevented by interviewing more accessible substitutes. Rather, interviewers must strive to interview every selected person. Training interviewers in nonjudgmental attitudes, careful question structure, and culturally appropriate wording are important strategies to reduce respondent self-presentation bias. Surveys on STIs, sexual behaviour, and HIV require special attention to issues of informed consent, anonymity, and confidentiality. The effect of the location of the interview (household or other settings such as clinics, workplaces, or community centers) on respondent's perception of privacy has not yet been adequately measured.

The lessons learned from previous validity and reliability checks in developing countries show that evidence is varied and that the acceptability of measurement errors may well depend on the objectives of the surveys. For example, a constant bias over time is less important for monitoring trends than for developing an appropriate intervention or making epidemiologic forecasts. Validity checks of different kinds are needed that are compatible with time and resources pressures in order to identify errors and biases and to be certain that behavioural changes are real and not due to the unreliability of reports. Triangulation is especially needed not only to validate the accuracy of responses but also to provide a context for the interpretation of quantitative indicators.

Techniques to Assess Reliability

Reliability usually refers to the ability of a method to give consistent results over many tests, repeated at different times. While low reliability always means low validity, high consistency of responses across several measurement may reflect a constant bias. Reliability may be directly assessed by test-retest measures, using the same instrument and method. It can also be assessed indirectly by examining internal consistency. Dare and Cleland recently reviewed five reliability studies conducted in various countries with retest subsamples of about 300 respondents at an interval of 2 to 6 weeks after the main survey8. Consistency varied not only according to specific variables and questions but also according to the characteristics of the study population. At the group level, however, reliability was acceptable for most of the key sexual risk behaviour factors.

SAMPLING STRATEGIES FOR MONITORING HIV RISK

As described in the preceding study, "Uses of Behavioural Data for Programme Evaluation," using repeated surveys to monitor trends in behaviours that put people at risk of contracting or passing on HIV infection and other sexually transmitted infections (STIs) is an important aspect of evaluation strategies for HIV/AIDS prevention and care programmes. Consensus has coalesced around the idea that monitoring risk behaviours ("behavioural surveillance") should be undertaken for both the general population and for selected subpopulations whose behaviours or life circumstances put them at risk for HIV transmission (sex workers, men who have sex with men, injecting drug users, mobile populations) or because of their vulnerability to risk (youth)1. Guidance about undertaking target group surveys and discussions of relevant indicators, questionnaire design, and validity and reliability issues are presented in other chapters of this study. Procedures for undertaking general population HIV risk behaviour surveys are described elsewhere. The method used to choose respondents or subjects is a crucial aspect of any survey effort. Indeed, the credibility of efforts to monitor trends in HIV/AIDS risk and protective behaviours on the basis of repeated surveys will depend as much as anything on the method(s) used to choose survey subjects. Because most of the groups of interest for HIV target group surveys are difficult to locate or enumerate, sampling presents a formidable challenge.

This study provides guidance on sampling for repeated surveys designed to monitor trends on HIV risk-related behaviours in key subpopulations. This study begins with a discussion of major sampling issues and problems for target group surveys. Two prototype designs that should cover most target group survey needs are described, followed by illustrative applications of the prototype designs. Sample size requirements for repeated target group surveys are then considered. The final section considers several related survey and sample design issues for sub-population surveys.

Major Issues

An important challenge in conducting meaningful target group surveys is to devise sampling plans that are both feasible and capable of producing unbiased estimates (or, more realistically, estimates with acceptably small levels of bias) for population subgroups that are not easily captured in conventional household surveys. First generation HIV risk behavioural surveys in target groups by and large resorted to informal or non-probability sampling approaches. However, recent efforts have attempted to put risk behaviour monitoring on a more solid scientific footing by adopting more rigorous sampling methods. Perhaps the central sampling issue to be addressed is the desirability and feasibility of using probability sampling methods in such undertakings. The major advantages of probability over non-probability sampling are twofold: It is less prone to bias, and it permits the application of statistical theory to estimate sampling error from the survey data themselves3. It is these features that make probability sampling methods the preferred choice whenever feasible. The major disadvantage is that a list or sampling frame is needed. While there are ways to make the task of developing sampling frames less costly and time consuming, it will nevertheless involve greater time and expense than would the adoption of a sampling approach not requiring a sampling frame. The primary attraction of non-probability sampling methods is that they are less time consuming and costly to implement. However, there are several important drawbacks. The first is the risk of sampling bias. Where a list of sampling units is not available from which to select a sample following fixed rules, there is the danger that certain types of subjects will be disproportionately included in and others disproportionately excluded from the sample. The second is the issue of replicability, which is of key importance for surveys intended to monitor behavioural trends over time. Where sample selection criteria are not defined in operationally precise terms such that they may be replicated in subsequent survey rounds, there is the danger that measured trends may be confounded by changes in sampling methodology. Finally, there is the problem that because such methods are not driven by statistical theory, there is no objective basis for assessing the precision or reliability of survey estimates.

In the final analysis, the issue reduces to one of the relative importance of "defensible" survey findings for the purposes for which the data are sought. In the event of unexpected findings, the use of non-probability sampling methods may leave a programme vulnerable to questions about the "representativeness" or "unbiasedness" of the data. This is not to say that in any particular undertaking, a survey based upon non-probability sampling methods will not produce the same results as a probability survey. There is, however, greater credibility risk associated with the use of non-probability sampling methods.

In view of the need for accurate information on behavioural trends for HIV/AIDS prevention programmes, a case may be made for moving from non-probability to probability sampling methods to the extent feasible. However, is probability sampling feasible for the population subgroups of interest for HIV/AIDS programmes? Although probability sampling is more demanding, recent experience indicates that with modest levels of technical support, several national HIV/AIDS programmes have been able to make the transition to the use of more rigorous sampling. As will be demonstrated in this study, the basic ideas of probability sampling may be extended in a fairly straightforward manner to cover most of the population subgroups of interest for HIV risk behaviour surveys. However, the use of probability sampling methods will not be feasible for some types of target groups, notably those whose members do not tend to congregate in fixed locations and for whom it is thus difficult to develop a sampling frame. For such groups, the use of non-probability sampling methods is the only alternative.

As a practical matter, sampling for target group surveys will require:

— the use of different sampling strategies for different target groups;
— the collection of data in non-household settings for most target groups;
— the use of conventional probability sampling approaches in non-conventional ways; and
— the occasional use of non-probability sampling methods (in situations where probability methods are infeasible).

Cluster Sample Design

The prototype probability sample design for subpopulation surveys is a two-stage cluster design. Adaptations on the basic design should satisfy the sampling requirements for a majority of target groups surveys.

Defining Clusters

Central to the extension of cluster sampling methods to surveys of difficult-to-enumerate population subgroups is a flexible definition of a "cluster." A cluster, or more precisely a primary sampling unit or PSU, is any aggregation of elements of interest (such as persons, households, or target group members) that can be unambiguously defined and used as a sampling unit from which to select a sample of elements of interest. Many readers will be familiar with the use of geographic areas as clusters or PSUs in household surveys. For the purposes of target group surveys, PSUs may be defined as any identifiable site or location where target group members congregate or may be found. .

Prototype Sampling Schemes

Two prototype sampling schemes for HIV target group surveys are described in this section. The first is an extension of conventional cluster sampling to groups who are difficult to enumerate. The second is a more rigorous form of snowball sampling known as targeted sampling.

Developing Sample Frames

A sampling frame is simply a list of subjects of interest for a particular survey or, in the event that such a list does not exist, a list of sites or locations where members of a target group of interest are known to congregate. Sampling frames are an integral part of probability sampling. Indeed, the applicability of probability sampling methods to HIV risk behaviour surveys hinges upon it being possible to construct meaningful sampling frames. Except for the case of youth (who may be covered through household surveys), sampling frame development for subpopulation surveys will require preliminary fieldwork to identify for use as PSUs the locations where members of target groups tend to gather. The process of gathering this information is known as ethnographic mapping, which simply means that basic ethnographic techniques are used to create the maps-specifically, participation observation, key informant interviews, and spending time "walking the community." Creating the sampling frame may only involve creating lists of sites. In other instances, it may be necessary to prepare sketch maps. The maps need not have precise dimensions and distances; rough drawings including such things as main streets, main features of the landscape or other identifiable features, and most importantly, main places where target group members "hang out" will suffice.

Occasionally, lists and maps of locations of key gathering points for target group members, such as brothels, bars, massage parlors, truck stops, hotels, recreation sites, schools, or other locations, may already exist. Sometimes, non-governmental organisations (NGOs) who have been working with a subpopulation may have already created maps of their catchment areas. It is important that sampling frames cover the entire geographic universe defined for a given survey effort and include the large majority of sites or locations where target group members congregate. If not, the resulting survey estimates will be prone to bias if the behaviours of target group members excluded from the possibility of selection for the survey differ from those who were surveyed. Where the creation of a sampling frame is infeasible for the intended universe for a survey effort, the only alternative under probability sampling is to restrict the universe to that for which it is possible to create a sampling frame.

Selecting Sample Clusters

Once a sampling frame of relevant PSUs has been created, unless the number of sites or locations is sufficiently small that they may all be covered in a given survey, a sample will need to be chosen. The recommended procedure for doing so will depend upon whether any information on the size of clusters (in other words, the number of target group members associated with each site or cluster) is available before the selection of sample clusters.

Statistically, the most efficient procedure is one in which PSUs or clusters are selected using systematic sampling with probability-proportional-to-size (PPS) at the first stage and a constant number of target group members chosen from each PSU at the second stage. Such a design results in a sample in which each target group member has the same overall probability of selection. This is known as a self-weighted sample. In addition to being relatively efficient in terms of sampling precision, this design eliminates the need to weight the data during analysis.

PPS selection should be used when establishments vary significantly in terms of numbers of sex workers associated with them; for example, when some establishments have five times or so as many sex workers as other establishments. Where the numbers of sex workers associated with establishments are roughly comparable, selecting clusters with equal probability will suffice. However, PPS selection requires that a sampling frame with measures of size (MOS) be available or developed before the sample is selected. A measure of size is simply a count or estimate of the number of elements, or target group members, associated with each PSU. Exact counts are not necessary for use as measures of size-rough approximations will suffice. Unless the errors in measures of size are quite large, the bias introduced into the survey estimates generally will be modest.

When measures of size for clusters are not available, sample clusters will have to be chosen with equal probability. Depending upon how sample elements are chosen at the second stage of sample selection, selecting PSUs with equal probability may result in sample elements having different probabilities of selection. In other words, the sample may be non-self-weighting, and it will be necessary to apply sampling weights to the data at the analysis stage if unbiased survey estimates are to be obtained.

Selecting Target Group Members Within Sample PSUs

In conventional cluster sampling, sample elements are chosen from a list of elements associated with each sample cluster using either simple random or systematic sampling. For many target groups, however, developing a relatively complete list of elements associated with each sample site is likely to be problematic.

Two alternative approaches to second stage sample selection are proposed. The first option, a quota sampling approach, entails interviewing target group members as they come into contact with sample sites or locations until a target sample size has been achieved. For example, a sample of truck drivers might be selected by interviewing all truck drivers who happen to appear at the truck stop until the target sample size has been achieved. Note that under this strategy, the length of time required to achieve the target sample size will vary depending upon the volume of contacts with sample sites.

Alternatively, a "take-all" strategy could be adopted in which all target group members who come into contact with a sample site during a specified data collection interval (for example, on a particular day or night) would be included in the sample irrespective of their number. The keys to the "take-all" strategy are that (1) data be collected at each sample site for the same amount of time at each site, and (2) data are obtained from all target group members that come into contact with each sample site during the designated data collection period. Thus, the "take-all" strategy is not recommended when large numbers of target group members congregate at the sites to be used as PSUs or when it is not possible for other reasons to capture all target group members who appear at sample sites during a specified data collection period. In such situations, the quota sampling approach is instead recommended. For the "take-all" strategy to be workable, it will be necessary to have at least rough estimates of the typical number of target group members associated with each site. This information is needed to determine both how many sites need to be included in the sample and how many interviewers need to be assigned to each site in order to "capture" all of the target groups members who come into contact with each site on the randomly chosen day.

Targeted Snowball Sampling

The primary role envisioned for non-probability sampling in target group surveys is as a substitute for probability methods in situations where the latter prove to be infeasible. This occurs largely in instances where constructing an adequate sampling frame of sites or locations where target group members congregate is not possible. Target groups for which non-probability sampling methods may have to be used include injecting drug users (IDU), some types of sex workers, and possibly men who have sex with men (MSM). The basic form of non-probability sampling recommended for target group survey efforts is a modified snowball sampling referred to as targeted sampling5. The basic idea in snowball sampling is to compensate for the lack of a sampling frame by learning the identities and/or locations of members of a given network of target group members through interviews with informants and other target group members themselves. Snowball sampling is an inherently iterative process. Typically, the data collection process begins by interviewing informants and target group members known to the researchers in order to learn the identities of other target group members. The researchers then contact these persons, collect the data, and obtain information on where additional target group members might be found. Leads from each wave of referrals are followed up until a sample of pre-determined size has been achieved. An important limitation of snowball sampling is that sample target group members are likely to provide information only on other target group members who are in their own social, economic, and/or sexual network. To the extent that risk-taking and/or protective behaviours differ across networks, this poses a potential bias problem for target group surveys. Research in San Francisco, California, for example, revealed the existence of social networks that differ in terms of race, ethnicity, and type of drug used, even in relatively compact geographic areas. Thus, in order for the snowball sampling approach to yield meaningful monitoring data, it is necessary to ensure that target group members from different networks in a given setting are included in the sample.

Targeted sampling is a combination of street ethnography, stratified sampling, quota sampling, and snowball or chain referral sampling. Watters and Biernacki5 describe this approach as being "a purposeful, systematic method by which controlled lists of specified populations within geographic districts are developed and detailed plans are designed to recruit adequate numbers of cases within each of the targets. While they are not random samples, it is particularly important to emphasize that targeted samples are not convenience samples. They entail, rather, a strategy to obtain systematic information when true random sampling is not feasible and when convenience sampling is not rigorous enough to meet the assumptions of the research design."

Three basic steps are involved in taking a targeted sample:

— initial geographic mapping;
— ethnographic mapping and stratification; and
— recruitment of quotas of target group members in specified subcategories through snowball sampling.

Applications of the Prototype Designs to Selected Target Groups

The following sections contain examples of how the various sampling designs described above may be used with sex workers, men who have sex with men, injecting drug users, and youth.

Sampling Frame Development

In most settings, at least some sex workers will work from fixed establishments, such as brothels, massage parlors, or bars. For sex workers who do not work from fixed establishments, city blocks, public parks, and other locations where sex workers congregate may be used as sample sites.

Once a list of sites has been created, it can be used to construct a sampling frame consisting of time-location segments, which are used as PSUs. To illustrate, suppose that preliminary research in a given setting revealed 20 commercial sex establishments. If establishments were open 7 days per week, a total of 140 PSUs would be formed (20 sites x 7 days). If sample PSUs are to be chosen with probability proportional to size, the listing or sampling frame of establishments should also include a measure of size for each PSU. The appropriate measure of size is the expected number of sex workers at a given site on a given day.

The rationale for doing this is to try to spread out the

sample over different times/days of the week in the event that sex workers with differing behaviours work on different days of the week. For example, it might be the case that "part-time" sex workers whose behaviours differ from "full-time" sex workers work only on weekends. To ensure an adequate distribution of sample PSUs with respect to such characteristics as geographic location and type of establishment, researchers typically order the sampling frame according to such factors. For example, commercial sex establishments might be ordered by first listing establishments located in the northwest quadrant of the city, followed by establishments in the southwest quadrant, and so on. Within each quadrant, establishments would be ordered by type of establishment. If two or more cities are included in a target group survey, geographic stratification could be accomplished by listing all establishments in the first city, then those in the second city, and so on.

Sex Workers

Domains and Stratification

An initial issue to be addressed in undertaking surveys of sex workers is whether different types of sex workers in a given setting differ with regard to risk-taking and protective behaviours. For example, in Senegal a distinction is made between registered and clandestine sex workers; in India, between brothel-based and freelance sex workers; in Kenya, between high- and low-paid sex workers; and in Thailand, between "direct" and "indirect" sex workers (namely, sex workers working in massage parlors or brothels versus those working as bartenders or waitresses in bars or restaurants who also engage in commercial sex). If behaviours are thought or known to differ, it would be advisable to treat the types of sex workers as separate survey domains. If not, then they can be treated as a single domain (although as separate sampling strata).

"Broker"—based Sex Workers

In some settings, sex workers who are not based in establishments may not congregate in public places, and thus, the cluster sampling approach described above will be infeasible. In India, for example, encounters with sex workers are sometimes arranged through "brokers." In other settings, arrangements are made by telephone. If a significant portion of the commercial sex trade operates in this fashion in a given setting, then probability sampling methods will not be feasible and the targeted snowball sampling approach will be necessary.

Selection of Sample Clusters and Sex Workers

Once the sampling frame has been developed, a sample of PSUs can be chosen either with probability-proportional-to-size or with equal probability, and a sample of sex workers using either a quota sampling or a "take-all" approach.

Injecting Drug Users (IDUs)

Of the groups to be covered by target group surveys, IDUs may well be the most difficult to survey. Among the problems likely to be encountered are difficulties in locating sufficient numbers of IDUs and in obtaining cooperation in responding to the survey. There is an absolute need to safeguard the identity, location, and confidentiality of anyone cooperating in the effort to obtain data from potential informants, as well as IDUs themselves.

With regard to sampling, IDUs may not congregate in sufficient numbers for a cluster sampling approach to be effective. However, in some settings it may be possible to identify areas of cities where higher than average concentrations of IDUs may be found. For example, in HIV/AIDS-related research in San Francisco, it has been feasible to use key informant interviews and consultations with police and medical authorities to identify neighborhoods or districts with significant numbers of IDUs. Even if a sufficient number of such areas can be identified, it will still be necessary to identify the different social networks operating. Accordingly, the targeted snowball sampling approach is likely to be the most feasible alternative in most settings.

Men Who Have Sex With Men (MSM)

Men who have sex with men (MSM) are difficult to enumerate in sample surveys. However, in many settings, MSM tend to congregate in certain types of establishments or locations (for example, certain bars, nightclubs, parks, or neighborhoods) in sufficient numbers that such locations may be used as PSUs for cluster sampling. In many settings, this may be the only feasible means of gathering behavioural data on MSM. It should be recognized, however, that because not all MSM frequent such locations, this approach is prone to bias to the extent that the behaviours of MSM who frequent such locations differs from those who do not. Alternatively, the targeted snowball sampling approach could be used. The proposed cluster sampling approach for MSM is quite similar to that used for sex workers who are not based in establishments. The initial step is the development of a sampling frame of locations where MSM congregate. In compiling the list of establishments, attention should be paid to ensuring that the frame covers all geographic parts of the survey universe and that all relevant networks are included, such as those defined by specific ethnic or socioeconomic characteristics.

Once a list of establishments/locations has been developed, time-location sampling units should be created for use as PSUs. For example, if 10 establishments or locations were identified and establishments were open 7 days per week, a total of 70 PSUs would be created. Note, however, that if preliminary research indicated that MSM tended to frequent such establishments only on certain nights, the sampling frame might be limited to such nights. The list of PSUs should be ordered geographically and by establishment type before sample selection.

Youth

Youth differ from the other groups that might be covered in target group surveys in that household surveys may be the preferred way to go about monitoring behavioural trends. Only youth who reside at school, who are institutionalized, or who have no fixed place of residence (for example, homeless or street children) would be excluded from the universe of a household survey. However, in some settings it may not be acceptable to survey youth at their place of residence about sensitive topics. If so, it will be necessary to identify segments of the general population of youth for whom it is feasible to locate and interview outside of their homes. For example, one might consider for inclusion as proxy groups youth in schools, youth working in the informal sector of the economy (such as street hawkers), and youth working in low-skill occupations in the formal sector (such as domestic workers or apprentices). Finally, special categories of youth, such as homeless or street children, might be considered.

Household Surveys of Youth

When household surveys are to be used to enumerate youth, the conventional two-stage cluster sample design proposed for general population surveys by WHO is the recommended sampling approach2. As this sampling scheme is well documented elsewhere, it will not be discussed here. However, a comment on the procedure used to select a sample of youth within sample PSUs is in order.

The preferred procedure is to first create a list or sampling frame of all households containing one or more youth located within each sample PSU, and then choose a sample of households using either simple random or systematic sampling. However, because creating complete lists of households with youth tends to be costly and time consuming, shortcut procedures are often used, which sometimes introduce substantial bias. A more robust shortcut method, referred to as the segmentation method, has seen increasing use in recent years. The basic approach is to divide sample clusters into smaller segments of approximately equal size, choose one segment at random from each cluster, and interview all youth found in households in the chosen segment. The advantages of this approach are twofold in that it (1) avoids the household listing operation, and (2) results in a self-weighting probability sample. The method is described in detail elsewhere9,10.

A key issue in household surveys of youth concerns the way in which sample youth who are not available to be interviewed should be handled. In some surveys, fieldworkers are instructed to merely substitute other respondents, such as in a neighboring household. For target group surveys of youth, this practice should be discouraged because of the potential bias that may be introduced. For example, youth who engage in high-risk behaviours may be more likely to live in single-parent households and/or to be at home less regularly, thus making it more difficult to locate them for a survey interview.

If such persons are systematically excluded from target group surveys, the survey data will underestimate the extent of risk behaviour. The recommended course of action is to require return visits ("call-backs") to each sample household in order to obtain an interview from each sample respondent.

School Surveys of Youth

In settings where a sizeable proportion of youth remain in school at the intermediate and secondary levels, conducting surveys in schools represents a cost-effective way of reaching youth. Two cluster sampling schemes for undertaking school surveys are described below. The first is for use when surveys can be conducted in school classrooms using self-administered questionnaires; the second is used when data collection has to take place outside of classroom settings.

The logistically simplest approach is to have students' complete self-administered questionnaires during class sessions. In addition, the low cost of self-administered questionnaires might enable data to be obtained for larger samples of students than will be feasible if personal interviews are used to collect the data. When "in-class" data collection is possible, a two-stage cluster sample design should satisfy most target group survey needs. Under this design, a sample of schools is first chosen from an ordered list of schools, then a sample of classes is chosen from an ordered list of classes in the identified sample schools, and data are gathered from all students in sample classes. Because measures of size (in this case, the number of school enrollees) are likely to be available before sample selection in most settings, schools should be chosen using systematic sampling with probability-proportional-to-size.

If in-class data collection in schools is not possible, it will be necessary to obtain data from students in non-classroom settings. Although it may be possible to schedule appointments with individuals or groups of students to be interviewed either before or after school, it also may be necessary to conduct intercept interviews with individual students at strategically chosen locations, such as outside of classrooms or in cafeterias, lunch rooms, or other common areas where students congregate.

Irrespective of the strategy used, it is important that steps be taken to ensure that the sample is sufficiently well spread out across students of different grades or levels. If students are to be interviewed as they enter or leave class, the classes or sections from which sample students are to be drawn should be chosen using a systematic-random selection procedure similar to that used in selecting classes or sections for in-class data collection.

Workplace Surveys of Youth

In order to obtain behavioural survey data on out-of-school youth, it is first necessary to determine where such youth may be found. One possibility is to interview youth at business establishments that typically employ youth. Examples of workplace sampling frames for youth in the informal sector include businesses employing apprentices, helpers of truck/bus/van drivers, and motorcycle taxi drivers.

As the types of businesses or occupations with significant numbers of youth are likely to vary from setting to setting, a generic sampling approach is proposed here. The recommended approach is a cluster sample design, with business establishments employing youth being chosen at the first stage of sample selection. As with most target group surveys, the sampling frame development process will begin with consultations with key informants and target group members themselves. The purpose of these consultations is to determine businesses that employ youth and the number of youth who are typically found at such businesses.

Once the sampling frame has been developed, a sample of workplaces can be chosen. If measures of size are available, workplaces should be chosen with probability-proportional-to-size and a fixed number of workers chosen per workplace using systematic sampling at the second stage of selection. However, if the number of workers present at workplaces varies significantly from day to day, it is instead recommended that workplaces be chosen with equal probability and the take-all strategy for selecting sample subjects within sample sites be used. Under this strategy, all youth workers present on the day and time each sample site is visited should be included in the sample. This approach eliminates the need to sub-sample workers in the event that the number present exceeds the target sample size for a given site, or conversely having to return to the site on another occasion in the event that the sample size quota is not met on a single visit. It also results in a self-weighting sample.

Surveys of Youth with No Fixed Residence

For youth who do not have a fixed place of residence, a modified cluster sampling approach in which neighborhoods, city blocks, public parks, and other locations where youth with no fixed residence are known to congregate are used as PSUs. The number of sites of PSUs to be chosen will depend upon how many youth are expected to be found per PSU per interval of fieldwork. If only small numbers of youth are typically found on a given day or night, more PSUs or clusters will need to be included in the sample to reach the target sample size. Alternatively, the same sites could be visited on more than one night, although this may well result in many duplicate interviews. Note, however, that if this strategy is followed, the number of nights that each site was visited needs to be documented so that the sampling weights can be adjusted accordingly. Additionally, if the number of sites where street youth congregate is small (for example, fewer than 10), it may be necessary to include all sites in the sample.

Mobile Populations

Individuals in mobile populations are of concern for HIV/AIDS programmes because they spend considerable periods of time away from home, and in many settings and cultures they tend to engage in casual sexual relationships and use the services of sex workers on a more frequent basis than is observed in the general population. In some cases, mobility may involve crossing national borders. Examples of mobile populations include transportation workers, merchants, and migrant laborers. The basic cluster sampling approach described above is easily extendable to these groups. The major variation lies in the nature of the sites or clusters to be used in cluster sampling.

Determining Sample Size Requirements

The primary objective of repeated behavioural surveys is to measure and compare changes in behavioural indicators over time. The size of the sample is a key design parameter in any survey because it is crucial in ensuring sufficient statistical power to detect and measure such changes. The sample size required per survey round to measure change on a given indicator will depend upon five factors:

— the initial or starting level of the indicator:

— the magnitude of change that evaluators wish to be able to reliably detect;

— the probability with which evaluators wish to be certain that an observed change of the magnitude specified did not occur by chance (that is, the level of significance);

— the probability with which evaluators wish to be certain that the actual change of the magnitude specified will be detected.

— the relative frequency with which persons with the characteristics specified in a given indicator may be found in the target group population.

The design effect (D) is the factor by which the sample size has to increase in order to produce survey estimates with the same precision as a simple random sample. It is based on the homogeneity or similarity within and between the clusters. In short, the greater the differences between the clusters compared to within the clusters, the greater the sample size must be to compensate for these differences. Assuming that the number of cluster sample sizes can be moderately small in a given survey (not more than 20-25 individuals), the use of a standard value of D = 2.0 should adequately compensate for the loss of accuracy resulting from two-stage sampling designs.

A table based upon this formula that permits readers to determine final sample sizes without having to perform calculations is provided in a Technical Appendix at the end of this study. The table provides sample sizes needed to measure changes in behavioural indicators of a magnitude of 10 and 15 percentage points for different initial values of a given indicator and for different combinations of significance (a) and power (ß). The sample sizes provided in the Appendix table are based on one-tailed values of Z1-a (one-sided significance test), assuming a rationale exists for anticipating the direction of change in behavioural indicators in settings where HIV/AIDS prevention interventions have been introduced. This will result in smaller sample sizes than if corresponding two-tailed z-score values of Z1-a/2 (two-sided significance test) were to be used. Two-tailed z-score values are appropriate when the direction of change cannot reasonably be predicted and/or if programmes wish to take a more cautious stance with regard to sample size requirements.

For some indicators, a second sample size computation step will be needed. Take, for example, the indicator "proportion of male vocational students who used a condom during their last encounter with a female sex worker." In this case, the first step in calculating the sample size required would be to determine how many students would be needed to measure a change in the proportion who used a condom during an encounter with a female sex worker during the previous year as described above-for illustrative purposes, say n = 200. However, because only students who had an encounter with a female sex worker in the last year are to be considered in this indicator, it will be necessary to determine how many students would have to be interviewed in order to find the required number of respondents who had sex with a female sex worker during the prior year. Computationally, the procedure is simple. One merely divides the required sample size calculated as described above by the estimated proportion of the target group that exhibited the required "qualifying" behaviour. For example, if 40 percent of male vocational students in a given setting are thought to have had sex with a sex worker in the last year, it would be necessary to interview n = 500 (= 200/.4) students to find n = 200 subjects needed to measure the desired indicator.

The more difficult part is anticipating what the appropriate underlying proportion would be. Here, other surveys or anecdotal information might be consulted for guidance. As there may be considerable uncertainty concerning these parameters, the general guidance is to err toward underestimating the proportion engaging in a given behaviour, as this will ensure a sufficient sample size for the main survey effort. For example, if it were thought that between 20 percent and 30 percent of students typically engage in sex with sex workers on an annual basis in a given setting, the 20 percent figure should be used in determining sample size requirements for target group surveys. The sample size requirements for any given target group survey will be the largest of the sample sizes calculated for the key indicators measured by the survey.

Determining the Magnitude of Change to Measure

One of the more important considerations in determining sample size requirements is the magnitude of change to be measured. The quantity (P2-P1) is the minimum change in a given indicator that successive target group surveys aspire to be able to measure accurately. Sample size requirements vary inversely with the magnitude of (P2-P1). For small values of (P2-P1), the required sample size may be quite large. For practical reasons, it is thus recommended that risk behaviour surveys not attempt to measure changes in behavioural indicators smaller than 10-15 percentage points. Attempts to measure smaller changes will likely exceed the resources available to most such efforts.

It should be emphasized that the magnitude of change in a parameter specified in sample size determination calculations may or may not correspond to programme targets with regard to the indicator in question. In some cases, a programme might have to accept measuring changes of larger magnitude than what they expect to achieve in a given period of time. This is because measuring changes of smaller magnitude may not be feasible. For example, where condom use in a given setting is only 5 percent, a programme might wish to measure a 5 percent increase in a 1-year period. However, they may have to be satisfied with measuring a 10 percent increase over a 2-3 year period instead. This is because the sample size required to detect a change of 5 percentage points may be larger than the available resources for survey-taking can support. In this case, the change parameter (P2-P1) might be set to 10 or 15 percentage points in determining sample size requirements, simply because this is all that is feasible. Even though the programme target of increasing condom use by 5 percentage points within 1 year may have been reached, it will not be possible to conclude statistically that the indicator has changed until a change of 10-15 percentage points has been realised unless, of course, additional resources can be found to support surveys with larger sample sizes. In other words, the sample size is too small to give the survey enough power to detect such a small change as statistically significant and to demonstrate that the programme actually had an effect on condom use.

Considering Statistical Power

A second key sample size consideration is that of statistical power. Unless sample sizes are sufficient to be able to detect changes of a specified size, the utility of repeated surveys as a monitoring tool is compromised. To illustrate, suppose we desire to be able to measure a change of 10 percentage points in the proportion of sex workers who always use a condom with their clients. We compare two pairs of hypothetical surveys taken 2 years apart: one with a sample size of n = 500 in each survey round and the other with a sample size of n = 200 per survey round. While both surveys might indicate the expected increase of 10 percentage points, this change may well not be statistically significant at a given level of significance based upon the surveys with sample sizes of n = 200. Thus, we would be forced to conclude that no meaningful change in this behaviour occurred over the study period, when, in fact, there was a real increase but it was not statistically significant. To ensure sufficient power, a minimum value of Z1-b of .80 should be used; .90 would be preferable where resources permit. Further guidance on determining sample size requirements for target group surveys is provided in Family Health International's *Guidelines for Repeated Behavioural Surveys in Populations at Risk of HIV12.*

Other Sample and Survey Design Issues

Retaining or Replacing Sample Sites or Clusters in Each

Survey Round

One of the key design issues in repeated surveys is whether to retain the same PSUs or clusters or choose a new sample of sites in each survey round. There are two advantages to retaining the same sample of sites or clusters. The first is that background characteristics and behaviours of individuals associated with particular sites tend to be correlated over time, and this factor can increase the statistical precision with which changes are measured. For example, sites such as brothels, bars, or truck stops may attract certain types of target group members and/or may encourage or discourage certain types of behaviours. The effect of this correlation is to reduce the standard error of survey estimates of change between the two survey rounds. Secondly, retaining the same sites reduces the sampling frame development work that needs to be done at the beginning of each survey round.

Balanced against this are several important disadvantages. Among these, the problem of resistance by site "gatekeepers" to repeated visits to the same sites and the loss of sites due to business failures loom especially large. In some settings, the sites where members of certain types of target groups congregate might change so rapidly over time that there is no choice but to construct a new sampling frame and select a new sample of sites in each survey round. Finally, retaining the same sites over an extended period of time does not allow for new sites or "pockets" of risk behaviour to be reflected in the behavioural survey monitoring data.

While a compromise strategy of retaining a fixed proportion of sites between any two successive survey rounds and replacing the remaining sample of sites with a new sample might be considered, the advantages of retaining even some sample sites over time in target group surveys are debatable. For one thing, it is unclear that the correlations on characteristics and behaviours over time will be as large for the types of sites used in target group surveys as is often found when residential areas are used as clusters in household surveys. Thus, the magnitude of gains to be realised by maintaining the same clusters is uncertain. The general recommendation, therefore, is to choose a new sample of sites in each survey round.

Dealing with Duplicate Observations

Irrespective of which sampling method is used, one problem that may occur is that of duplicate observations. Duplicate observations may arise because some target group members are associated with more than one PSU. For example, sex workers may work at more than one location, or truck drivers may use more than one truck stop during the course of fieldwork for a survey. There is thus a possibility that the same target group member might be interviewed twice or possibly more.

The statistically correct way to deal with this problem is to adjust the sampling weights to account for the fact that some target group members had more than one opportunity to be included in the sample for a given survey round. However, the recordkeeping, statistical, and data processing requirements of doing so are likely to be beyond the resource capacity in most applications.

A more feasible, but less technically satisfactory solution would be to screen out potential duplicate observations by inquiring whether sample target group members had already been interviewed during the period of survey fieldwork, and not conducting interviews with respondents answering yes. If this approach were adopted, appropriate screening questions would have to be added at the beginning of the survey questionnaires used. A third option is to do nothing.

Except when the total population of a target group of interest is very small, the probability of encountering a sufficient enough number of duplicate observations in a given survey round to introduce serious bias is likely not large enough to worry about.

Dealing with Insufficient Numbers of Target Group Members at Sample Sites

In many of the sampling schemes described above, a number of decisions are driven by an expected number of target group members at each site during a specified time interval. What should be done if, during the course of fieldwork, researchers find that the actual number of target group members is substantially lower than expected?

Two options are available. The first is to return to sample sites for additional intervals of data collection. The second is to select a supplementary sample of PSUs. Returning to sample sites for an additional interval of data collection is the less desirable option for two reasons. First, if the expected daily volume of target group members were a serious overestimate, returning to the same sites would be an inefficient way of increasing the sample size. Secondly, sampling additional cases per PSU would increase the precision of survey estimates less so than sampling additional PSUs. What should be done in cases where all PSUs are already included in the sample, and it is thus impossible to choose more PSUs? In this situation, the only alternative is to visit sample PSUs for longer intervals than had been originally planned.

What should be done if even after repeated visits to all PSUs, it is still not possible to reach the target sample size? The answer to this question depends upon the reason why it was not possible to reach the target sample size. One possible cause is that the sampling frame was incomplete.

In such a case, one option would be to update the sampling frame and choose a supplementary sample of PSUs of sufficient size to enable the target sample size to be reached. Alternatively, a lower-than-planned sample size could be accepted for the current survey round, and more resources could be put into sampling frame development in subsequent survey rounds in which larger sample sizes would be used (larger sample size in subsequent survey rounds can offset the effects of sample size deficit in earlier rounds). In Nepal, one approach to dealing with this problem was to inquire from successfully interviewed establishment-based sex workers about any friends who worked at the same establishment but had not been present during the times that data were being collected for the target group survey. These leads were then followed up and included in the sample as having been sampled from the "referring" establishment. Such an approach should be used cautiously, however. In the Nepal case, researchers found that a number of the leads were in fact not sex workers, but friends of the sex workers who were nominated so that the sex worker could collect the incentive offered for identifying other sex workers. In the final analysis, it may have been preferable to accept a lower than expected sample size. A final note on the problem is that in some instances, there may simply not be enough target group members in the population. In such cases, the key issue is whether there is sufficient justification for doing surveys for the target group.

Ensuring Replicability Through Documentation

Given the difficult sampling problems posed by HIV/AIDS target group surveys, it is important that steps be taken to make the resulting data as unbiased and sampling plans as replicable as possible. Of crucial importance is that a thorough documentation of sampling plans and adopted selection criteria is prepared to enhance the replicability of data collection efforts over time. This is especially important where probability sampling methods are not used, as the credibility of estimated trends in behaviours over time depends very heavily upon whether a convincing case can be made that identical sampling and survey methods were used across repeated survey rounds. Being able to demonstrate that constant sampling procedures were used adds considerably to the credibility of such estimates. Monitoring trends in HIV risk behaviours through periodic surveys presents some formidable sampling challenges. At the heart of these problems is the fact that many of the population subgroups or target groups that may be of interest for behavioural surveillance or monitoring are difficult to capture in conventional household surveys. In this study, we have described in some detail two approaches to sampling for risk behaviour surveys in key HIV target groups. The first approach extends the basic principles of cluster sampling in ways that should be both applicable and feasible for most target groups. The second approach, a more rigorous form of snowball or chain referral sampling, is recommended for use when the development of any type of meaningful sampling frame of sites where target group members congregate is infeasible. Applications of these two strategies to the key HIV target groups were presented in the study. By providing guidance on more rigorous sampling methods, we hope the validity and quality of risk behaviour surveillance data can be greatly improved. We acknowledge, however, that the use of these more rigorous sampling approaches in undertaking repeated risk behaviour surveys is still in the testing stage. While recent experience suggests that the recommended approaches are feasible, further verification is required. Applications planned in a wide variety of settings over the next few years should provide further guidance on how relatively rigorous sampling methods for such survey undertakings might be adapted to meet field realities.

6

Hospital Rehabilitation Service and Support Group: A Case Study

Rehabilitation services are needed by people who have sustained severe injury, often due to trauma, a stroke, an infection, a tumor, surgery, or progressive disease. A pulmonary rehabilitation programme is often appropriate for people who have chronic obstructive lung disease. People whose bodies become severely weak after prolonged bed rest (for example, because of a heart attack or surgery) are also in need of rehabilitation. Physical therapy, occupational therapy, and the treatment of any pain and inflammation are the focus of rehabilitation.

The need for rehabilitation crosses all age groups, although the type, level, and goals of rehabilitation often differ. People with chronic impairments, often older people, have different goals, require less intensive rehabilitation or a longer period of rehabilitation, and need different types of therapy than do younger people. For example, the goal of an older person with severe heart failure who has had a stroke may be to restore the ability to perform as many self-care activities (eating, dressing, bathing, transferring between a bed and a chair, using the toilet, controlling bladder and bowel) as possible. The goal of a younger person who has had a heart attack or been in a car accident is often to restore full, unrestricted function. Nonetheless, age alone is not a reason to alter goals or the intensity of rehabilitation; the presence of disease and limitations, however, may be. Intensive rehabilitation that involves several components, such as physical therapy, occupational therapy, and speech therapy, usually requires continued sessions of one-on-one training for weeks to be of benefit. Sometimes, more immediate health concerns must be attended to before rehabilitation can be addressed. To initiate a formal rehabilitation programme, a doctor writes a referral (similar to a prescription) to a physiatrist (a doctor who is board-certified in rehabilitation medicine), an occupational or physical therapist, or a rehabilitation center. The referral establishes the goals of therapy, a description of the type of illness or injury, and its date of onset. The referral also specifies the type of therapy needed, such as ambulation training (help with walking) or training in activities of daily living (for example, help with eating, dressing, grooming, or toileting). Where the rehabilitation takes place varies according to the person's needs. Care in a hospital or rehabilitation center may be necessary for people with severe disabilities. In such settings, a rehabilitation team provides care. Along with the doctor or therapist, this team may include nurses, psychologists, social workers, other health care practitioners, and family members.

The rehabilitation team or therapist establishes specific short-term goals for each of the person's problems, which may include restricted range of motion, an uncoordinated gait, and the inability to open a jar or feed himself. The person is encouraged to achieve each short-term goal, and the team closely monitors the person's progress. The goals of therapy may be changed if the person is unwilling or unable (financially or otherwise) to undergo lengthy rehabilitation. Setting a long-term overall goal at the beginning helps people understand what can be expected of rehabilitation and where they can expect to be in several months. People who require less care, such as those who can transfer from bed to a chair or from a chair to a toilet, can often obtain rehabilitation services in an office or at home. In such cases, however, family members or friends must be willing to participate in the rehabilitative care process. Providing rehabilitation at home with the help of family members is highly desirable, but it can be physically and emotionally taxing for all involved. Sometimes, a visiting physical therapist or occupational therapist can help with home care. Regardless of the severity of the disability or the skill of the rehabilitation team, the final outcome of the rehabilitation process depends on the person's motivation. In some cases, a person may prolong recovery in order to gain attention from family or friends

Changi General Hospital: Asthma Support Group

The Asthma Support Group at Changi General Hospital counsels patients with Bronchial Asthma, Chronic Obstructive Lung Disease (COLD), Cor Pulmonate, Chronic Obstructive Pulmonary Disease (COPD), Bronchitis and other medical conditions relating to asthma. Our healthcare professionals are always ready to assist you.

The Asthma Support Group also conducts community health talks on asthma care. We aim to increase awareness in the community, by achieving the following objectives:

- To educate patients on the basic patho-physiology of Bronchial Asthma
- To provide information on the principles of Asthma Management
- Teach patients to recognize the warning signs of severe asthma

— To assess inhaler techniques- teach and demonstrate correct techniques and return demonstration by patients

— Motivate and encourage the use of inhalers

— Teach patients to use and monitor peak flow readings

— Monitor response to treatment and advice on allergen avoidance

— Teach effects of asthma medication

— Educate and counsel family members.

Patients and families are kindly requested to bring their inhalers and case sheet to the counselling sessions. Asthma education protocol is used as a standard way in documentation and guide to counselling and educating the patients. The basic patho-physiology of asthma and aims of treatment are taught, along with symptom recognition and warning signs of worsening asthma. Our support group also explains the use and care of inhalers and asthmatic devices such as a spacer or aerochamber, and Peak Flow Monitoring. They also discuss allergy trigger factors, asthma medications and an Emergency Management Plan, in the event of a severe asthma attack. Improvement of the home environment is also addressed, as environmental factors play an important role in asthma management. Coping with asthma emotionally, psychologically and physically is difficult, but with the assistance and advice from our support group, we aim to make asthma management simple and worry-free. The CGH Breast Support Group was created specially to help women who are newly diagnosed with breast cancer or who have undergone mastectomy (removal of the breast). Our goal is to provide you with the emotional support and information you need to cope and to understand your condition.

Our support group is run by a committed group of counsellors from the hospital. They are nurses, doctors and medical social workers who provide compassion, advice and a listening ear to patients.

The activities of the Changi General Hospital Breast Support Group include:

— Explanation of pre and post operative management
— Complete psychological and emotional support
— Advice on physical recuperation
— Understanding of your fear of an altered body image
— Teaching of exercises to enable full recovery of shoulder movements
— Care of operation wound
— Care of an affected arm
— Advice on how you can cope better when undergoing chemotherapy and radiotherapy.
— Provide recommendation on when, where and how to obtain prosthesis

  and wigs
— Provide information on other resources available in Singapore, such as the Breast Cancer Foundation and the National Cancer Centre.

The CGH Breast Support Group conducts various programmes and events during the year. This includes support and social programmes for members of the support group and public forums.

Understand Your Cancer- Live A Positive Life!

What Is Breast Cancer?

Breast cancer occurs when some cells in your breast

grow abnormally. Cancer cells differ from normal cells in several ways. They vary in size, shape, and divide more quickly. The cells sometimes move into other areas of the body. There are different types of breast cancer. Your doctor will inform you on the type of cancer you have.

Renew Your Self-Image

You may have a lot of mixed feelings about your body. You may be concerned that a removal of a breast will somehow leave you feeling less feminine or less attractive to others.

Determine Your Treatment

After the results of your biopsy are known, you may have to make a decision to have a mastectomy with your surgeon.

Cope With Your Diagnosis

Put your own needs first. You may want privacy and/or the support of family, friends or our CGH Breast Cancer Support Group.

How is Screening Done?

Mammography is currently the most effective method of screening for breast cancer, especially in women between 50 and 65 years. It is a low dose x-ray imaging technique that produces pictures of the breast tissue. A radiographer takes the x-rays and the films are interpreted by our radiologists.

Recovery in the Hospital

It is important to perform the recommended exercises after your surgery, as these exercises help to regain the motion and strength in your arm and shoulders. The counsellor from the Support Group will instruct you on these.

Prepare for Surgery

A counsellor from our CGH Breast Support Group will help prepare you psychologically and emotionally before and after surgery.

Take Care of your Affected Arm

Lymphedema is the swelling of the arm which occurs when the normal flow of fluid in the arm is reduced. Performing the recommended exercises may help to reduce lymphedema.

Learn to Cope with Your Feelings

Talking about breast cancer with your loved ones may be hard. Your family and friends may not know what to say or do.

Breast Cancer Screening

Breast Cancer Screening helps to detect breast cancer at an early stage before there are any changes in the breast are noticeable to you or your doctor.

Early detection and treatment of breast cancer results improves the survival outcome. Not all women with breast cancer need to have a mastectomy. If the cancer is discovered at an early stage, the need for a mastectomy is low.

Do You Need Support?

Our Breast Support Group at Changi General Hospital is always available to answer any questions you may have and to clarify any doubts.

How is Mammography Done?

A female radiographer at our Department of Radiology will conduct your mammogram. You will be required to change into a hospital robe. You will be asked a few questions about your medical history and your breasts may be examined before the mammogram.

The radiographer will position your breast between 2 plastic plates and when the x-ray is taken, the plates will compress the breast firmly for a few seconds. This is necessary to ensure good visualisation of the breast tissue.

Preparing for Mammography

On the day of the mammography, do not use any powder, deodorant or lotion on the chest, breasts or armpits, as it may affect the quality of the mammogram.

For your convenience, we suggest you wear two piece outfit instead of a dress as you will need to undress to the waist.

Please bring along any previous mammogram films. This will help our radiologist to detect any changes from previous mammograms.

When Should I do a Mammogram?

The American Cancer Society (ACS) recommends that women should have mammograms when:

Around 40 years: First mammogram

40-49 years: Every 1 or 2 years

Over 50 years: Every year

Women at higher risk may be required to have mammograms more frequently or start at an earlier age.

If you have particularly sensitive breasts, schedule your mammogram for the week after the start of your period. Your breasts will be less tender then, so you will feel less discomfort during the mammogram.

Hospital Procedure

At the wards, our stoma care nurses provide consultation relating to the management of stomas. Patients with stomas may be referred as early as the first post-operative day. This is to prevent the occurrence of potential complications, such as skin excoriation. At CGH, patients and their relatives will be given the name of the stoma care nurse who attended to them. Patients and family are encouraged to contact their nurse if they require further assistance after discharge.

What Happens after the Mammography?

The films will be reviewed and interpreted by a radiologist. Occasionally, we need to conduct additional tests to achieve a full assessment. Please do not be alarmed if you are contacted, as it does not always mean that there are any abnormalities in your breasts.

Additional tests that may be conducted are:

— Special mammogram views

— Ultrasound - uses sound waves to determine if the growth is a solid mass or fluid-filled (cyst)

Whether you have just developed diabetes or have been a diabetic patient for some time, quite often you will be concerned about sugar control, lipid control and blood pressure control.

Our Changi General Hospital Diabetes team can help equip you with knowledge on self-care survival skills for diabetes, so that you can cope better with diabetes in day-to-day living. Regular talks on diabetes are held for patients, and topics discussed in these classes include meal planning, anti-diabetic medications, foot care and exercise. CGH also runs a Skills for Life: Diabetes programme.

The CGH Diabetes team has also published a book "Diabetes Totally Uncovered" in English and Chinese. This book is filled with real life experiences and practical tips on how to manage diabetes.

Changi General Hospital's Stoma Care Support Group offers counselling and support to patients and their families, before and during their rehabilitation process after stoma surgery. We understand the importance of having the knowledge and skills look after a stoma patient.

The Stoma Care Support Group aim to:

- Advise and demonstrate the way to take care of the stoma and peristomal skin area, draining wounds and fistula
- Provide guidance to patients and family with regards to caring for and living with a stoma
- Co-ordinate training sessions for medical professionals with patients on stoma care

NUTRITIONAL SUPPORT

There is a consensus that nutritional support should be routinely provided to intensive care unit (ICU) patients. Hospitalized patients with malnutrition (macronutrient and/or micronutrient deficiency) suffer from increased infectious morbidity, prolonged hospital stays, and increased mortality. Moreover, even those hospitalized medical and surgical patients without antecedent malnutrition are typically subjected to stress, infection and impaired organ function, resulting in a hypercatabolic state. Often these patients are unable to meet their caloric needs, as they are either too sick or physically unable to ingest food. Although strong evidence demonstrates that providing nutritional support for such patients results in improved clinical outcomes, the optimal method of delivery, timing of administration, and specific formulation requires further research.

Prevalence and Severity of the Target Safety Problem

Malnutrition in hospitalized patients often goes

unrecognized. Early studies reported a prevalence of malnutrition in 30-50% of hospitalized patients. A later study revealed that up to 40% of patients were malnourished at the time of their admission. The majority of these patients continued to be nutritionally depleted throughout their hospital course. These patients are also at a greater risk for the development of severe malnutrition than those patients whose nutritional status was adequate at the time of admission. Unfortunately, there is no single, readily available measure of malnutrition that is both sensitive and specific in critically ill patients. Most studies have used body mass index (BMI=weight (kg)/height (m)) and/or anthropometry (measuring skin fold thickness) to assess patients' nutritional status. BMI alone is not a sensitive indicator of protein-energy malnutrition as it does not distinguish between depletion of fat or muscle. In a large number of studies, malnutrition has been defined as a BMI £ 20 kg/m and a triceps skin fold thickness (TSF) or mid-arm muscle circumference (MAMC) <15 percentile. Patients with a BMI of £ 18 and £ 16 kg/m with anthropometric measurements below the 5 percentile were considered to have moderate and severe malnutrition respectively. Weight loss exceeding 10% of ideal body weight (IBW) also suggests malnutrition.

Practice Description

There are several ways to provide nutritional support to patients in the ICU. Enteral nutrition (EN) can be administered via transoral, transnasal, or percutaneous transgastric routes, or by surgical jejunostomy. Total parental nutrition (TPN) is generally used when the enteral route is either inaccessible or its use is contraindicated. It is also used as a supplement to enteral feeding if adequate nutrition is not possible via the enteral route alone. The total caloric requirement of critically ill patients can be estimated or directly measured. Calorimetry, although accurate, is not practical in the clinical setting as it is costly, time consuming, and requires technical skill. It is also unclear that exactly matching energy input with energy expenditures improves patient outcomes. Therefore, a pragmatic approach is to attempt administration of 25 kilocalories per kilogram ideal body weight per day for most patients. The total caloric daily requirement should be administered in a fluid volume consistent with the patient's needs (usually 1mL/kcal). Protein sources should comprise 15-20% of the total daily calorie requirement. The generally accepted amount of protein is between 1.2 and 1.5 g/kg per day, except in severe losses such as burns. Glucose should comprise 30-70% of the total calories and fats 15-30%.

Study Design

The field of nutritional support can be divided into several basic areas of investigation. First, research has evaluated whether nutritional support is of benefit to malnourished critically ill patients. Second, studies have compared the impact of EN versus TPN on patient outcomes. Further investigations have looked at the timing of administering nutritional support. Lastly, recent research has focused on the type of EN, specifically considering whether immune-enhancing formulas (immunonutrition) improve outcomes. At least 26 randomized controlled trials (RCTs) have compared the use of TPN to standard care (usual oral diet plus intravenous dextrose), and one meta-analysis reviewed these studies. A different meta-analysis specifically reviewed the use of TPN in surgical patients. A systematic review with meta-analysis (duplicated in the other publications) included evaluation of 6 randomized trials in surgical patients that compared the benefits of early enteral nutrition with standard care. Numerous randomized controlled trials have compared EN to TPN. Three RCTs of surgical patients evaluated the merits of early enteral feeding postoperatively. A few studies have compared EN delivered into the stomach versus into the small bowel (jejunum). Several randomized controlled trials have studied the effects of using immunonutrition and we found 2 meta-analyses of immune-enhancing enteral supplementation in critically ill patients after trauma, sepsis or major surgery.

Opportunities for Impact

Providing nutritional support has the potential to significantly reduce several clinically relevant endpoints (e.g., infectious complications, hospital stay, mortality). However, even when malnutrition is recognized, adequate nutrition is often not delivered. Prescription of optimal enteral nutrition to meet energy requirements ranged from 76% to 100% in a prospective survey of 5 ICUs in the United Kingdom. Another study of enteral nutrition among patients receiving no oral nutrition in medical and coronary care units at 2 US university-based hospitals, documented that physicians ordered only 65.6% of daily goal requirements and only 78.1% of this was actually delivered. A recent prospective study of both enteral and parenteral nutrition in a French university-affiliated ICU found that physicians prescribed only 78% of the mean caloric amount needed by patients, and only 71% of this was effectively delivered. Efforts targeted at increasing physician awareness of the problem and early delivery of appropriate nutrition may improve patient outcomes.

Study Outcomes

The majority of studies reported Level 1 outcomes including infectious complications and mortality. Some measured hospital length of stay (Level 3) as well. Several studies evaluating immunonutrition reported its effects on surrogate outcomes such as wound healing. Studies evaluating immediate enteral nutrition in burn patients have also used surrogate markers. Animal studies have assessed the effects of immunonutrition on gastrointestinal physiology as well as wound strength.

Evidence for Effectiveness of the Practice

Nutritional supplementation in hospitalized patients may reduce mortality and is associated with weight gain. However, there are no randomized controlled trials comparing supplemental nutrition to starvation in critically ill patients. Research does show that patients not receiving any nutritional support for more than 2 weeks postoperatively have a much higher complication and mortality rate than patients receiving TPN or some short-term glucose administration. A large body of research in the past 2 decades has focused on determining the ideal type and method of delivery of nutritional support.

A meta-analysis comparing supplemental TPN to standard care (oral diet as tolerated and intravenous dextrose) found no effect on mortality (relative risk (RR) 1.03, 95% CI: 0.81-1.31). There was a trend toward a lower complication rate among those receiving TPN (RR 0.84, 95% CI: 0.64-1.09), but this is due mainly to benefit among malnourished patients. There are no data from randomized controlled trials to support the use of supplemental TPN among patients with an intact gastrointestinal tract ("If the gut works, use it"). Several studies have evaluated the use of supplemental EN in surgical patients. These studies often used surrogate outcomes, but one randomized double-blind trial of early EN versus standard diet as tolerated following surgery found fewer total complications (26.7% vs. 63.3%, p=0.009), fewer infectious complications (6.7% vs. 46.7%, p<0.001) and a trend towards a reduction in hospital length of stay (8 vs. 11.5 days, p=0.08) with early EN. Based on this evidence, early EN is recommended in critically ill surgical patients. There is no specific research evaluating the benefits of supplemental EN in critically ill medical patients, but results from research in surgical patients appear to be applicable. In animal studies, EN promotes gut motility, reduces bacterial translocation, prevents mucosal atrophy and stimulates the secretion of IgA that helps to reduce infectious complications. There is also evidence that EN improves nutritional outcomes and results in greater wound healing. A review of 5 trials studying postoperative EN found no significant reduction in morbidity or mortality. However, a recent study of patients with non-traumatic intestinal perforation and peritonitis found there to be a total of 8 septic complications in the early EN group versus 22 in the control group ($p<0.05$).

Multiple studies comparing use of EN to TPN in critically ill medical and surgical patients demonstrate that EN is safe, less expensive, and results in similar or better outcomes. Among patients with acute severe pancreatitis, those fed enterally had fewer total complications (44% vs. 75%, $p<0.05$) and fewer septic complications (25% vs. 50%, $p<0.01$). In numerous studies of surgical patients, EN also appears to be more effective than TPN. A study of patients undergoing total laryngectomy revealed no difference in mortality or infectious complications. However, the patients who received TPN had a longer length of stay (34 days vs. 11 days, $p<0.05$). In another study of patients with abdominal trauma, those fed enterally had significantly fewer septic complications (15.7% vs. 40%, $p<0.02$). A meta-analysis combining data from 8 prospective randomized trials found that 18% of patients receiving EN developed infectious complications compared with 35% in the TPN group ($p=0.01$). Of note, EN may not be preferred to TPN in head-injured patients. In a study of patients with head trauma there appeared to be no significant difference in relation to infectious outcomes and mortality between EN and TPN. However, patients fed enterally had a trend toward a higher incidence of aspiration pneumonia (32% vs. 13%, p=0.11), though no difference in overall infections and mortality. The effects of preoperative TPN have been evaluated in 13 prospective randomized controlled trials of patients undergoing surgical resection of a gastrointestinal tumor. Combining the data from these studies reveals a modest reduction in surgical complications (approximately 10%) in those patients receiving TPN. This benefit appears to be due entirely to significant reduction in surgical morbidity among patients who are severely malnourished. Therefore, preoperative TPN may be of benefit in severely malnourished patients undergoing major gastrointestinal surgery, but EN should be used instead, if possible. The use of postoperative TPN has been evaluated in 8 prospective randomized trials of patients undergoing gastrointestinal surgery. Patients in the combined TPN group experienced an increased rate of complications (27.3% vs. 16.0%; p<0.05). Thus, routine use of postoperative TPN in this setting is not recommended.

Since enteral administration is the preferred method of nutritional support, additional research has focused on the utility of early administration of EN to severely ill surgical patients. In animal studies early EN is associated with greater wound strength after abdominal surgery. In burn patients immediate EN was associated with a decrease in catecholamines and glucagons, and improved nitrogen balance compared to delayed EN. A prospective randomized controlled study evaluated the effect of immediate jejunal feeds in patients with major abdominal trauma. The overall complication rate was similar in both groups, but 9 patients in the control group developed postoperative infections versus 3 in the EN group (p<0.025). Although other studies do not show a change in outcomes, based upon this data it is reasonable to begin EN as soon as possible in surgical patients. More research is needed to evaluate the necessity of administeri

ADVANCE PLANNING FOR END-OF-LIFE CARE

Physicians and other healthcare workers have long struggled with decisions regarding care for patients at the end of life. An important component of this care involves assessing and understanding patient preferences for care through ongoing discussions with competent adult patients and/or their family members or surrogates. Advance care planning protects patient autonomy and helps to assure that their health and medical treatment wishes are implemented. Good communication at the end of life can also help patients achieve closure and meaning in the final days of their life. Over the past 20 years, public consciousness regarding planning for end-of-life care has been raised through several seminal court cases, such as those involving Karen Ann Quinlan and Nancy Cruzan. These cases and the public interest they helped engender led to legislation promoting patients' rights to determine their care at the end of life. For example, Natural Death Acts (statutes passed by state legislatures that assert a person's right to make decisions regarding terminal care) have helped promote the use of living wills (described below). In addition, in 1990 the federal Patient Self-Determination Act (PSDA) was passed by Congress to encourage competent adults to complete advance directives. The PSDA requires hospitals, nursing homes, health maintenance organisations, and hospices that participate in Medicare and Medicaid to ask if patients have advance directives, to provide information about advance directives, and to incorporate advance directives into the medical record.

Advance directives are any expression by a patient intended to guide care, should they lose their medical decision making capacity. Although both oral and written statements are valid, the added effort required to complete written statements gives them greater weight. In addition to their use when patients lose competence, advance directives also help patients consider the type of care they would want in the future, even if they retain decision making capacity. Advance directives have legal validity in almost every state.

There are 2 principal forms of written advance directives: living wills and durable powers of attorney for healthcare. A *living will* is a document that allows an individual to indicate the interventions he or she would want if he or she is terminally ill, comatose with no reasonable hope of regaining consciousness, or in a persistent vegetative state with no reasonable hope of regaining significant cognitive function. A *durable power of attorney for healthcare* (DPOA-HC) is a more comprehensive document that allows an individual to appoint a person to make healthcare decisions for him or her should he or she lose decision making capacity.

Prevalence and Severity of the Target Safety Problem

Respecting patient preferences regarding end-of-life care requires a well-coordinated approach. Problems can arise in both documenting patient preferences and ensuring that preferences are available and respected at the time they are needed. In addition, inadequate communication with patients can compromise the goal of respecting patient preferences for end-of-life care through a variety of mechanisms.

Failure to Document Preferences

The PSDA was a legislative solution designed to increase rates of completed advance directives. Although there was initial hope that PSDA would markedly increase rates of advance directive documentation, by the early 1990s it was clear that the impact was small. At that time, a large multicenter randomized trial, the Study to Understand Prognoses and Preferences for Outcomes and Risks of Treatments (SUPPORT), was undertaken to improve advance care planning. SUPPORT represents one of the largest and most comprehensive efforts to describe patient preferences in seriously ill patients, and to evaluate how effectively patient preferences are communicated. SUPPORT cost 28 million dollars and enrolled 9100 seriously ill patients. In SUPPORT, a trained nurse facilitator provided prognostic information to patients and medical staff, discussed patient preferences with patients and families, and facilitated communication between patients and physicians. Neither the PSDA legislation nor the SUPPORT intervention had major impacts on the documentation of patients' preferences regarding end-of-life care. Teno et al reported on the documentation of advance directives at 3 points: before PSDA, after PSDA, and after the SUPPORT intervention. The percentage of patients with an advance directive was unchanged in all 3 groups, but documentation of those directives increased at each stage, from 6% to 35% to 78% in the SUPPORT intervention group. Despite this increase in documentation, only 12% of patients with an advance directive had talked with a physician when completing the document and only 25% of physicians were aware of their patients' advance directives. SUPPORT found that only 23% of seriously ill patients had talked to their doctors about their wishes concerning cardiopulmonary resuscitation (CPR) and that patient-physician discussions and decisions were uncommon even in seriously ill patients whose death was predictable. Another study that surveyed elders in community settings found that the vast majority (81%) stated their desire to discuss their preferences with their physicians if they were terminally ill, but only 11% had done so. As these studies demonstrate, patients often want to talk about death and dying but expect physicians to bring up the issues.

Ensuring that Preferences are Available and Respected

Even when advance directives are prepared, studies show they often do not change interventions at the end of life. Advance directives are frequently not available, recognized or applied, nor do they help reduce hospital resource use. There are multiple reasons why advance directives may go unrecognized. Admitting clerks may fail to document or incorrectly document the status of a directive on admission to the hospital. Patients and families often do not inform the hospital physician or admitting clerk about their advance directives, or fail to bring documentation to the hospital. In one survey of 200 patients, only 18% had filled out an advance directive and of these, 50% had secured the only copy in a safety deposit box! A copy of the advance directive is often not transferred from the nursing home to the hospital on admission. In a study by Morrison, physicians documented advance directives or discussions with appointed proxies about treatment decisions in only 11% of admission notes.

Although the goal of advance directives is to ensure that patients receive treatment that is consistent with their preferences, to date there is no evidence that documenting advance directives leads to this outcome. In SUPPORT, there was no evidence that increasing the rates of advance directives resulted in care more consistent with patients' preferences. This finding was concordant with a study of nursing home patients and their family members regarding preferences for aggressive treatment at the end of life. There, 25% of patients received care that was inconsistent with their previously expressed wishes. The problem may not be the substance of advance directives *per se*, but rather in the manner in which clinicians approach them. Physicians may be hesitant to initiate discussions of advance directives with patients, especially early in the course of an illness.

Despite these shortcomings, advance directives remain the best available approach for helping patients plan future care. These discussions, difficult as they are, help ensure that patients receive care consistent with their values and goals, spare the patient inappropriate interventions, and help maintain dignity during the dying process.

Physician Communication

In order to improve the quality of end-of-life care, physicians need to effectively communicate with their patients and understand their preferences for care. Several studies have documented imperfections in physician-patient communication. Several studies have demonstrated that physicians often misunderstand or are unaware of their patients' preferences for care. Furthermore, physician prediction of patients' preferences for resuscitation are no better than random. In summary, the published literature demonstrates significant problems in all areas crucial to advance care planning and ascertainment of patient preferences, transmission of information to appropriate care settings, and respecting those preferences. The provision of unwanted end-of-life care is an adverse event that can potentially be avoided by the implementation of effective patient safety practices.

Opportunities for Impact

Patients with chronic or life-limiting illnesses make up a large proportion of the adult primary care population. Almost three-quarters of the 2.3 million Americans that die each year are 65 years of age or older. By the year 2030, people older than 65 will compromise 20% of the total population (70 million people), compared with 13% in 1994. Today's average life expectancy is 75.5 years, and the leading causes of death are heart disease, cancer and stroke. Data from 1995 estimated that these causes accounted for 62% of all deaths and 67% of deaths for those age 65 and over. The overall picture is of an aging population, with many individuals living for several decades (often with chronic diseases) after the possibility of death becomes more than theoretical. Support documented serious problems with terminal care. Physicians did not implement patients' refusals of interventions. When patients wished to forgo CPR, a do not resuscitate order was never written in about 50% of cases. While 90% of Americans say they want to die at home, 4 out of 5 die in a hospital or other healthcare facility. The SUPPORT study showed that only 35% of the study patients had an advance directive. These patients had an approximate six month mortality rate of 50%. Physicians and the public also commonly overestimate the effectiveness of CPR. In reality, in-hospital cardiac arrests have a survival rate of about 15%. For patients over 65 the survival rate is about 10-11%, and 3.5% for patients over age 85. Elderly nursing home patients with out-of-hospital arrest only have 1-2% survival. Studies have shown that when patients are aware of the real survival rates for CPR, they are less likely to desire this intervention.

Evidence for Effectiveness of the Practice

Documenting Preferences and Ensuring that they are Available and Respected

A Physician Order form for Life-Sustaining Treatment (the POLST)

In the mid-1990s, a task force of ethicists and clinicians at the Oregon Health Sciences University developed a new Do Not Resuscitate (DNR) order form called POLST (Physician Orders for Life-Sustaining Treatment). POLST is a comprehensive two-page order form that documents a patient's preference for life-sustaining treatments. The form is designed to record a patient's wishes clearly and simply. Tolle et al examined the extent to which POLST ensured that nursing home residents' wishes were honored for DNR orders, and for hospital admission only if comfort measures failed. None of the 180 patients who completed POLST received CPR, ICU care, or ventilator support, and only 2% were hospitalized to extend life.

The study subjects had low rates of transfer for aggressive life-extending treatments and high levels of comfort care. Since 1995, more than 220,000 copies of POLST have been distributed throughout the state. Data from 1999 suggest, albeit circumstantially, that this initiative may be working. In 1996, Oregon's in-hospital mortality rate was 31%, compared with the national average of 56%. Lee et al studied the effectiveness of POLST in a Programme of All-Inclusive Care for the Elderly (PACE) in Portland, Oregon. They retrospectively reviewed POLST instructions for each of the 58 participants and whether or not each of the treatments addressed by the POLST was administered in the final 2 weeks of life. The POLST specified DNR for 50 participants (93%); CPR use was consistent with these instructions for 49 participants (91%). The participants also designated the level of care they preferred as either comfort care, limited, advanced, or full intervention. Interventions administered were at the level specified in only 25 cases (46%), with less frequent deviations in antibiotic administration, administration of IV fluids, and placement of feeding tubes. The investigators concluded that the POLST effectively limits the use of some life-sustaining interventions, but that further investigation is needed into the factors that lead physicians to deviate from patients' stated preferences about other treatments.

Ascertaining Preferences in the Outpatient Setting

As with other forms of computerized decision support, computer-generated reminders for primary caregivers can increase the rates of discussion of advance directives and completion of advance directive forms among elderly outpatients with serious illnesses. Dexter et al performed a randomized, controlled trial to test the effectiveness of computerized reminders. The participants were 1009 patients and 147 primary care physicians in an outpatient setting. Physicians that received computer-generated reminders that recommended discussion of one or both of 2 types of advance directives were compared with physicians who received no reminders. Physicians who did not receive reminders (controls) discussed and completed advance directives in only 4% of the patients On the other hand, physicians who received both types of reminders discussed (24%) and completed (15%) advance directives significantly more frequently.

The Portability of Advance Directives between Hospitals and Nursing Homes

Ghusn et al retrospectively studied the relationship between inter-institutional communication and continuity of advance directives from hospital to nursing home settings. Having a hospital discussion about advance directives or having a hospital DNR order were associated with a higher rate of advance directive discussions in nursing homes. Hospital DNR orders were continued for 93% of patients discharged to the hospital-affiliated nursing home and 41% of patients discharged to the community nursing home. Specific communication of hospital DNR status to the receiving nursing homes was associated with better continuity of DNR orders. The authors concluded that completing advance directives before patients are discharged to nursing homes, communicating advance directives to the receiving home, and providing follow-up discussions at the nursing home might improve the continuity of advance directives between hospitals and nursing homes.

Administrative Initiatives to Ascertain Preferences on Admission to Hospital or Nursing Home

In addition to POLST, some medical centers have developed admission order forms to document patient preferences regarding end of life. These forms require healthcare personnel to inquire about advance directives, resuscitation preferences, artificial fluids and nutrition, etc. This approach, promoted by the passage of the PSDA, may be effective in promoting provider-patient discussions about end-of-life wishes and prevent unwanted treatments. However, there are no data documenting the effectiveness of this strategy.

Practices to improve physician-patient communication and physician understanding of patient preferences

Training for Physicians

Physician education is an attractive way to improve end-of-life care. Physicians often do not communicate about advance care planning because many have not been taught the relevant communication skills and have learned them only through personal experience. A study by Tulsky et al revealed that when physicians discussed end-of-life issues with their patients, they spoke twice as much as they listened and did not routinely explore patients' values. Until recently, training for healthcare providers in palliative care and respecting patient preferences, and materials to support such training, were inadequate. For example, recent studies have demonstrated that most medical and nursing textbooks insufficiently cover end-of-life care issues. Increasingly, resources (including textbooks, palliative care journals or journal series, Web sites and training programmes) are filling this educational void. The American Medical Association has developed an extensive physician training programme titled Education for Physicians on End-of-Life Care (EPEC). This curriculum teaches fundamental skills in communication, ethical decision making, palliative care, pain and symptom management, and other end-of-life treatment issues. The Robert Wood Johnson Foundation initiative, "Last Acts," is another ambitious effort to educate both patients and providers.

Other educational training programmes exist for physicians and students as well. Physicians can receive formal training by attending conferences on decisions near the end of life, case management meetings regarding individual patients, and seminars on communication skills with individual feedback to physicians on their performance. Physicians with expertise in this area often conduct seminars to educate physicians. Buckman and Lo have developed guides for specific end-of-life discussions, such as breaking bad news and the act of active listening and empathy. As attractive as these educational programmes are, none have been studied for their impact on changing practice or outcomes. Although common sense might tell us that such programmes are likely to be effective, the generally unimpressive relationship between professional education and outcomes or process change provides grist for uncertainty pending formal effectiveness studies.

Hospitalist Systems

Hospitalist physicians may improve end-of-life care in hospitals. Hospitalists, by virtue of their large inpatient volumes, should become increasingly facile with ascertaining patient preferences regarding end-of-life care. Hospitalists have a unique opportunity to approach patients, since an admission generally signals either a worsening of the patient's current condition or a new diagnosis. The hospitalist may have more time to spend with patients and is available over consecutive hospital days to answer any questions. A routine discussion of advance directives by hospitalists can help improve the quality and efficiency of patient care. On the other hand, patients may have a long-standing trusting relationship with their primary care physicians, and may have expressed their wishes to this physician prior to hospitalisation. This possibility highlights the importance of hospitalist-primary care provider communication, particularly concerning end-of-life issues. One retrospective chart review study of 148 patients dying at a community teaching hospital has examined the impact of hospitalists on end-of-life care. In this study, patients cared for by hospitalists were significantly more likely to have had a documented family meeting (91% vs. 63% for patients of community-based primary physicians). About two-thirds of patients in both groups requested limitations in the level of care by the time of death. Of these, patients of hospitalists were significantly less likely to have documented pain, dyspnea, or anxiety in the 48 hours prior to death (57% vs. 75%). Whether these differences reflect differences in the quality of care, the completeness of documentation, or underlying patient differences requires further study. Although the hospitalist movement holds promise for improving end-of-life discussions, more research is needed to determine whether this promise will be met.

Palliative Care Services

Specialized palliative care programmes have become increasingly common in the healthcare system. Physicians and other healthcare providers, including nurses, social workers, chaplains, and others are available to coordinate care and provide consultation for terminally ill patients in hospices, hospitals, nursing homes or patient's homes. The palliative care service also plays an important role in fostering communication among providers, patients, and families. Data regarding effectiveness are lacking.

Other Locally Successful Advance Care Planning Programmes

Individual programmes to implement patient preferences have emerged around the country. Limited data suggest that they may be effective, and bear further examination as to their portability to other programmes and settings and their durability over time.

"Respecting Your Choices" Program: Gundersen Lutheran Medical Center in La Crosse, Wisconsin has worked on community-wide programmes to improve advance care planning with an initiative called "Respecting Your Choices." This programme used patient and family education, community outreach, education for non-medical professionals, standard training sessions, and standard methods for documenting and tracking advance directives. Hammes et al reported that 85% of patients in the intervention group had written advance directives at death, executed on average 1.2 years before death. Of these directives, 95% were in the medical record. Virtually all patients (95%) reported that the interview process was meaningful. The patients felt that they benefited from improved communication with loved ones and with healthcare providers.

Dayton VA Initiative: The Dayton (Ohio) VA Medical Center aimed to increase the number of veterans who participated in advance care planning. VA patients and their families received a patient education booklet and a video on advance care planning. The VA also developed discussion guidelines for providers, initiated an advance care planning clinic, and initiated a bereavement support group. In a 12-week period, advance care planning discussions and follow-up increased from about 15% percent of charts to almost 90%.

"Let Me Decide" Program: Molloy et al examined patient satisfaction with decision making and healthcare costs after systematically implementing an advance directive programme in nursing homes. The "Let Me Decide" programme included educating staff in local hospitals and nursing homes, residents, and families about advance directives and offering competent residents or next-of-kin of mentally incompetent residents an advance directive. The researchers reported that systematic implementation of this programme reduced hospitalisations and aggressive care for nursing home patients who did not want that level of intervention. It also reduced utilisation of healthcare services without affecting satisfaction or mortality.

End-of-Life Education for the Public

Extensive public awareness and educational programmes are necessary to create a foundation for successful end-of-life conversations in patients with advanced illness. Broadcasts, such as the PBS-Bill Moyers special "On Our Own Terms," may help the public appreciate the experience of terminal illness, and the complex choices that are faced. Such presentations may encourage viewers to discuss how they might manage a similar situation, and explore their own fears and concerns about dying. There are no data regarding the effectiveness of public education to improve advance care planning.

Comment

Preventing unwanted aggressive care at the end of life requires active communication between provider and patient, and effective strategies to transfer information regarding preferences seamlessly across care venues. The dominant strategy to improve care in this area over the past 20 years has been the promotion of advance directives. Although the enthusiasm for advance directives has not been matched by evidence of their effectiveness, SUPPORT and other studies have renewed public concern and prompted providers and policy makers to reexamine advance care planning and strive to improve it. Although we have found evidence of several potentially promising strategies (perhaps the most promising of which is the POLST form), the inevitability of death and the importance patients place on improving end-of-life care point strongly to the need for further research in this area.

Costs and Implementation

Estimating the cost of ascertaining and respecting patient preferences is difficult since improvements in this area may require major changes in the structure of the healthcare system. Institutional barriers, the culture of medicine, patient attitudes, time constraints physicians face with office visits may all play a role in implementation and may inhibit change. Barriers to implementation include complacency on the part of the physician and patient, fear of political controversy, diffused responsibility, and absence (or perverse) financial incentives for providers and institutions. The surprising ineffectiveness of the SUPPORT intervention, which cost over 28 million dollars, demonstrates how difficult it is to make major improvements in this area. Nevertheless, improving our ability to respect patient preferences is valuable in its own right and may ultimately prove to be cost-effective, since some patients will choose to forego high technology and expensive care at the end of life. Medical care at the end of life consumes 10% to 12% of the total healthcare budget. An estimated 40% of the Medicare budget is spent during the last 30 days of life. Some have posited that increased use of hospice and advance directives and lower use of high-technology interventions for terminally ill patients will produce significant cost savings. However, the studies on cost savings from hospice and advance directives are not definitive. The 3 randomized trials of hospice and advance directives use show no overall savings, but the authors of a review suggest that the studies were either too small for confidence in their negative results or their intervention and cost accounting are flawed. In the absence of a definitive study, the existing data suggest that hospice and advance directives can save between 25% and 40% of healthcare costs during the last month of life, but far less (and perhaps nothing) in the 3-12 months before death. Although, these savings are less than most people anticipate, they do indicate that hospice and advance directives should be encouraged because they certainly do not cost more and they provide a means for patients to exercise their autonomy over end-of-life decisions. Finally, several of the promising interventions described above (e.g., the POLST intervention), are relatively inexpensive. For example, 500 POLST forms can be ordered from Oregon Health Science University's Web site for less than $100, although the cost of implementing the POLST programme is unknown.

Bibliography

Auerbach AD, Pantilat SZ, Wachter RM, Goldman L. Processes and outcomes of end-of-life care in a voluntary hospitalist model. *J Gen Intern Med* 2001; 16:115.

Basta L, Plunkitt K, Shassy, R, Gamouras G. Cardiopulmonary resuscitation in the elderly: Defining the limits of appropriateness. *Am J Geriatr Cardiol* 1998; 7:46-55.

Broadwell A, Boisaubin, EV, Dunn, JK, Engelhardt, HT. Advance directives on hospital admission: a survey of patient attitudes. *South Med J* 1993; 86:165-8.

Buckman R KY. *How to Break Bad News: A Guide for Health Care Professionals*. Baltimore, MD: Johns Hopkins University Press; 1992.

Christakis N, Iwashyna TJ. Attitude and self-reported practice regarding prognostication in a national sample of internists. *Arch Intern Med* 1998; 158:2389-95.

Covinsky KE, Fuller JD, Yaffe K, Johnston CB, Hamel MB, Lynn J, et al. Communication and decision-making in seriously ill patients: findings of the SUPPORT project. The Study to Understand Prognoses and Preferences for Outcomes and Risks of Treatments. *J Am Geriatr Soc* 2000; 48:S187-93.

Danis M, Southerland LI, Garrett JM, Smith JL, Hielema F, Pickard CG, et al. A prospective study of advance directives for life-sustaining care. *N Engl J Med* 1991; 324:882-8.

Dexter P, Wolinsky, FD, Gramelspacher, GP, Zhou, ZH, Eckert, GJ, Waisburd, M, Tierney, WM. Effectiveness of computer-generated reminders for increasing discussions about advance directives and completion of advance directive forms. A randomized, controlled trial. *Ann Intern Med* 1998; 128:102-10.

Donaldson M, Field, MJ. Measuring quality of care at the End of Life. *Arch Intern Med* 1998; 158:121-28.

Ebell MH, Becker LA, Barry HC, Hagen M. Survival after in-hospital cardiopulmonary resuscitation. A meta-analysis. *J Gen Intern Med* 1998; 13:805-16.

Emanuel EJ. Cost savings at the end of life. What do the data show? *JAMA* 1996; 275:1907-14.

Emanuel LL, von Gunten, C.F., Ferris, F.D. *The Education for Physicians on End-of-Life Care (EPEC) Curriculum*; 1999.

Ethics manual. Fourth edition. American College of Physicians. *Ann Intern Med* 1998; 128:576-94.

Gamble ER, McDonald PJ, Lichstein PR. Knowledge, attitudes, and behaviour of elderly persons regarding living wills. *Arch Intern Med* 1991; 151:277-80.

Ghusn H, Teasdale, TA, Jordan, D. Continuity of do-not-resuscitation orders between hospital and nursing home settings. *J Am Geriatr Soc* 1997; 45:465-69.

Hammes BJ, Rooney BL. Death and end-of-life planning in one midwestern community. *Arch Intern Med* 1998; 158:383-90.

Hanson LC, Tulsky JA, Danis M. Can clinical interventions change care at the end of life?. *Ann Intern Med* 1997; 126:381-8.

Jaret P. *Leading Patients in End-of-Life Decisions.* Hippocrates; 1999. p. 33-37.

Jonsen AR SM, Winslade WJ. *Clinical Ethics: A Practical Approach to Ethical Decisions in Clinical Medicine*. Fourth ed. New York, NY: McGraw-Hill; 1998.

Kurent J. *Death and Dying in America: The need to improve End-of-Life Care* Carolina Healthcare Business; 2000:16-19.

Larson DG, Tobin DR. End-of-life conversations: evolving practice and theory. *JAMA* 2000; 284:1573-8.

Lee M, Brummel-Smith, K, Meyer, J, Drew, N, London, MR. Physician orders for life-sustaining treatment (POLST): outcomes in a PACE programme. Programme of All-Inclusive Care for the Elderly. *J Am Geriatr Soc* 2000; 48:1219-25.

Lo B, McLeod GA, Saika G. Patient attitudes to discussing life-sustaining treatment. *Arch Intern Med* 1986; 146:1613-5.

Lo B, Quill T, Tulsky J. Discussing palliative care with patients. ACP-ASIM End-of-Life Care Consensus Panel. American College of Physicians-American Society of Internal Medicine. *Ann Intern Med* 1999; 130:744-9.

Lo B. Improving care near the end of life. Why is it so hard? [editorial; comment]. *JAMA* 1995; 274:1634-6.

Lynn J SJ, Kabcenell A. Beyond the Living Will: *Advance Care Planning for All Stages of Health and Disease. Improving Care for the End of Life: A Sourcebook for Health Care Managers and Clinicians*. Oxford University Press; 2000. p. 73-90.

McPhee S, Rabow, MW, Pantilat, SZ, Markcwitz, AJ. Finding our way—perspectives on care at the close of life. *JAMA* 2000; 284:2512-13.

Molloy DW, Guyatt GH, Russo R, Goeree R, O'Brien BJ, Bedard M, et al. Systematic implementation of an advance directive programme in nursing homes: a randomized controlled trial. *JAMA* 2000; 283:1437-44.

Morrison RS, Olson E, Mertz KR, Meier DE. The inaccessibility of advance directives on transfer from ambulatory to acute care settings. *JAMA* 1995; 274:478-82.

Muldoon MF, Barger SD, Flory JD, Manuck SB. What are quality of life measurements measuring? *BMJ* 1998; 316:542-5.

Pantilat SZ, Alpers A, Wachter RM. A new doctor in the house: ethical issues in hospitalist systems. *JAMA* 1999; 282:171-4.

Rabow M, Hardie, GE, Fair, JM, McPhee, SJ. End-of-life care content in 50 textbooks from multiple specialties. *JAMA* 2000; 283:771-8.

Teno JM, Licks S, Lynn J, Wenger N, Connors AF, Jr., Phillips RS, et al. Do advance directives provide instructions that direct care? SUPPORT Investigators. Study to Understand Prognoses and Preferences for Outcomes and Risks of Treatment. *J Am Geriatr Soc* 1997; 45:508-12.

Tolle SW, Tilden VP, Nelson CA, Dunn PM. A prospective study of the efficacy of the physician order form for life-sustaining treatment. *J Am Geriatr Soc* 1998; 46:1097-102.

Tulsky JA, Fischer GS, Rose MR, Arnold RM. Opening the black box: how do physicians communicate about advance directives?. *Ann Intern Med* 1998; 129:441-9.

Index

A

B

C

D

E

F

G

H

I

K

L

M

N

O

P

Q

R

S

T

U

V

W

Z